HOW TO COPE WITH YOUR
CHILD'S ALLERGIES

DR PAUL CARSON (B.A., M.B., B.CH., B.A.O., D.F.P.A.) holds an Asthma and Allergy clinic as part of his private practice in Dublin. He graduated from Trinity College, Dublin, in 1975 and spent six years working in Australia and England before returning to Ireland in 1983. He is a regular contributor to the *Irish Medical Times*, *Woman's Way*, *U-Magazine* and the Healthfax Press Agency in London. A series that he wrote on childhood asthma was syndicated to a number of provincial British newspapers and attracted much interest. In addition to writing, he lectures regularly to both doctors and the general public on asthma and allergic conditions. He is currently organizing a major survey on asthma among school children in Dublin.

MAURA THORNHILL, as well as catering for the needs of her allergic children, works as a health professional in a Dublin hospital.

GW00492571

Overcoming Common Problems Series

The ABC of Eating
Coping with anorexia, bulimia and
compulsive eating
JOY MELVILLE

Acne
How it's caused and how to cure it
PAUL VAN RIEL

An A–Z of Alternative Medicine
BRENT Q. HAFEN AND KATHRYN J.
FRANDSEN

Arthritis
Is your suffering really necessary?
DR WILLIAM FOX

Birth Over Thirty
SHEILA KITZINGER

Body Language
How to read others' thoughts by their gestures
ALLAN PEASE

Calm Down
How to cope with frustration and anger
DR PAUL HAUCK

Common Childhood Illnesses
DR PATRICIA GILBERT

Coping with Depression and Elation
DR PATRICK McKEON

Curing Arthritis Cookbook
MARGARET HILLS

Curing Arthritis – The Drug-free Way
MARGARET HILLS

Depression
DR PAUL HAUCK

Divorce and Separation
ANGELA WILLANS

Enjoying Motherhood
DR BRUCE PITT

The Epilepsy Handbook
SHELAGH McGOVERN

**Everything You Need to Know about Contact
Lenses**
DR ROBERT YOUNGSON

**Everything You Need to Know about Your
Eyes**
DR ROBERT YOUNGSON

Everything You Need to Know about Shingles
DR ROBERT YOUNGSON

Family First Aid and Emergency Handbook
DR ANDREW STANWAY

Fears and Phobias
What they are and how to overcome them
DR TONY WHITEHEAD

Feverfew
A traditional herbal remedy for migraine and
arthritis
DR STEWART JOHNSON

Fight Your Phobia and Win
DAVID LEWIS

Fit Kit
DAVID LEWIS

Flying Without Fear
TESSA DUCKWORTH AND DAVID
MILLER

Goodbye Backache
DR DAVID IMRIE WITH COLLEEN
DIMSON

Guilt
Why it happens and how to overcome it
DR VERNON COLEMAN

How to Bring Up your Child Successfully
DR PAUL HAUCK

How to Control your Drinking
DRS W. MILLER AND R. MUNOZ

How to Cope with Stress
DR PETER TYRER

Overcoming Common Problems Series

How to Cope with your Nerves
DR TONY LAKE

How to Cope with Tinnitus and Hearing Loss
DR ROBERT YOUNGSON

How to Do What You Want to Do
DR PAUL HAUCK

How to Cope with your Child's Allergies
DR PAUL CARSON

How to Enjoy Your Old Age
DR B. F. SKINNER AND M. E.
VAUGHAN

How to Interview and Be Interviewed
MICHELE BROWN AND
GYLES BRANDRETH

How to Love and be Loved
DR PAUL HAUCK

How to Say No to Alcohol
KEITH McNEILL

How to Sleep Better
DR PETER TYRER

How to Stand up for Yourself
DR PAUL HAUCK

How to Start a Conversation and Make Friends
DON GABOR

How to Stop Smoking
GEORGE TARGET

How to Stop Taking Tranquillisers
DR PETER TYRER

If Your Child is Diabetic
JOANNE ELLIOTT

Jealousy
DR PAUL HAUCK

Learning to Live with Multiple Sclerosis
DR ROBERT POVEY, ROBIN DOWIE
AND GILLIAN PRETT

Living with Grief
DR TONY LAKE

Living with High Blood Pressure
DR TOM SMITH

Living Through Personal Crisis
ANN KAISER STEARNS

Loneliness
DR TONY LAKE

Making Marriage Work
DR PAUL HAUCK

Making the Most of Middle Age
DR BRICE PITT

Making the Most of Yourself
GILL COX AND SHEILA DAINOW

Making Relationships Work
CHRISTINE SANDFORD AND WYN
BEARDSLEY

Meeting People is Fun
How to overcome shyness
DR PHYLLIS SHAW

No More Headaches
LILIAN ROWEN

One Parent Families
DIANA DAVENPORT

Overcoming Tension
DR KENNETH HAMBLY

The Parkinson's Disease Handbook
DR RICHARD GODWIN-AUSTEN

Second Wife, Second Best?
Managing your marriage as a second wife
GLYNNIS WALKER

Self-Help for your Arthritis
EDNA PEMBLE

The Sex Atlas
DR ERWIN HAEBERLE

Six Weeks to a Healthy Back
ALEXANDER MELLEBY

Solving your Personal Problems
PETER HONEY

Overcoming Common Problems Series

Overcoming Common Problems

HOW TO COPE WITH YOUR CHILD'S ALLERGIES

Dr Paul Carson

B.A., M.B., B.CH., B.A.O., D.F.P.A.

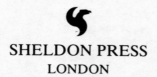

SHELDON PRESS
LONDON

First published in Great Britain in 1987 by
Sheldon Press, SPCK, Marylebone Road, London NW1 4DU

British Library Cataloguing in Publication Data

Carson, Paul
 How to cope with your child's allergies.——
 (Overcoming common problems)
 1. Pediatric allergy
 I. Title   II. Series
 618.92'97   RJ386

 ISBN 0–85969–529–8
 ISBN 0–85969–530–1 Pbk

Typeset by Deltatype Ltd, Ellesmere Port, Cheshire
Printed in Great Britain by
Richard Clay Ltd, Bungay, Suffolk

To my wife, Jean,
for the encouragement
and to all my young patients, for the inspiration

Contents

Preface

Allergic illnesses are on the increase in children, and allergies may be just as significant as infections as causes of ill health. It is a sad fact that many children suffer needlessly because of the current tendency to attribute the cause of illness to infection rather than to allergy.

Until recently, asthma, eczema, and hay fever were the main conditions accepted as due to allergy. However, doctors now recognize that a much wider group of common childhood illnesses have an allergic basis. In addition, the role of foodstuffs in causing many of these ailments has been firmly established.

Research into this relationship between diet and allergy has made health professionals far more aware of the extent of the problem, and identified the specific foods involved. Surprisingly, the main culprits turn out to be those substances which children consume regularly – milk, egg, wheat, chocolate, various types of soft drink and so on. These products surface time and again as being involved in a number of children's ailments, including asthma, eczema, migraine, hyperactivity, urticaria, colitis and even epilepsy. Not only can such foods cause symptoms when taken in their usual form (as is the case, for instance, with milk products) but they may also cause problems when they have been processed (as with, say, wheat in breakfast cereals, flour, cakes, etc.).

In this book you will read which common – and not-so-common – childhood illnesses are due to allergy and how they can be dealt with. You will learn what are the signs to look for in your child which might suggest an allergic basis to any persistent health problems. There are guidelines on allergy prevention and treatment, with specific diets suitable for individual conditions. In addition, there is a separate section written by the mother of an allergic child. She offers advice on dietary routines and includes some of her own low-allergy recipes. Finally, there are

1

success stories to help give you hope and encouragement should you be struggling with the management of an allergic child. The number of allergic disorders may be rising, but with careful treatment they can be alleviated. By using the information in this book you should be able to keep on top of these problems should they arise in your children.

Dr Paul Carson

1

The Allergic Conditions
of Childhood

Kevin was born in February 1982 after a normal, healthy pregnancy. His mother breast-fed him for eight months and then he was weaned on to a milk formula. Within days of starting on this formula, problems developed. He became irritable and cross, and began to bring back most of his feeds. At the end of the first week he developed a patchy red rash on his face, started to wheeze and had a very snuffly nose. He also appeared to have colic and diarrhoea.

The health visitor suggested trying a different formula, but this made no difference. At this point, Kevin's breathing became very distressed. Moreover, the patchy red rash had spread to involve the body and limbs. In desperation, Kevin's mother asked for an interview with a paediatrician at the local hospital. He suspected the child was allergic to the formula milk feeds, and admitted him to hospital for investigation.

While in hospital, Kevin was put on an intravenous drip and taken off all feeds for twenty-four hours. He settled quite quickly, and soon looked less miserable. He was then weaned gently back on to bottle feeds. This time, however, the formula was soya-based and caused none of the previous symptoms. At this early stage in Kevin's recovery, a special test was performed where a small piece of his bowel was examined under a microscope. It was found to be abnormal.

Within ten days of being put on the soya formula the child was showing a remarkable improvement: he had clearer skin, a settled chest and no colic. Also, he was more contented, less irritable and free from diarrhoea. A repeat bowel sample taken some weeks later showed that the lining was now normal. This more or less confirmed the diagnosis of a cow's milk allergy, but the paediatrician wanted to put Kevin back on milk once more to see if his symptoms returned. Not surprisingly, the child's mother refused: she had seen him suffer enough and was quite

3

satisfied with the diagnosis.

At the follow-up examination two months later, the paediatrician explained to Kevin's parents how an allergy to milk had been responsible for the child's difficulties. In particular, he pointed out that each separate symptom was almost certainly due to the milk allergy and would not recur while the child stayed off all milk products. He advised a milk-free diet for the next twelve months, at the end of which a review would be made to evaluate the possibility of reintroducing milk into Kevin's diet. The paediatrician suggested that while the child might well grow out of the milk allergy at some point, it was important that this should not be put to the test too soon.

Kevin, in fact, has not yet grown out of his milk allergy. On each occasion when milk has been introduced he has developed many of the same problems that were noted in hospital. In all probability he will react adversely to milk products for many years to come.

This rather dramatic story shows the difficulties allergy problems can pose for children and how time-consuming the management of these can be. Obviously, not every allergic child will show such severe responses – in many cases these are mild and of little consequence. However, the correct interpretation of Kevin's various problems was vital to his subsequent recovery. Had the symptoms affecting his skin, chest, nose and bowels been treated individually, he might have been prescribed drops for the nose, creams for the rash and two different syrups for the wheeze and diarrhoea. As it turned out, all that was required was the removal of the milk formula.

The role of allergy in children's ailments is no new discovery. What is new, though, is the recognition of the wide range of conditions that can be caused by allergy. Recent studies confirm that migraine, hyperactivity and epilepsy may have an allergic basis, with diet playing an important part in their management. These 'new' allergies can now be added to the list of well-known and accepted allergic conditions which include asthma, eczema and hay fever.

As Kevin's story shows, reactions due to allergy can have

effects throughout the body, producing a variety of symptoms. In his case the cause was milk, but for many children other substances are involved, such as household dust, various types of pollen or animal danders (a mixture of fur/hair, scale and urine).

Considering each of the body systems in turn, the following medical conditions of children are known to often have an allergic basis:

	Condition	Symptom(s)
Eyes	Conjunctivitis	Itchy, red eyes
Ears	Serous otitis media	Deafness, fullness in ear
Nose	Rhinitis	Itchy, runny nose
	Polyps	Blocked nose
	Post-nasal drip	Catarrh
Throat	Itchy palate	Itch along roof of mouth
Sinuses	Sinusitis	Feeling of pressure over sinuses
Lungs	Asthma	Wheeze, coughing, shortness of breath
Skin	Eczema	Red, itchy, weeping rash
	Urticaria	Red, bubbly, itchy weals
	Angio-oedema	
Nervous system	Migraine	Headaches, nausea
	Epilepsy	Convulsions
	Hyperactivity	Over-active, impulsive etc. behaviour
	Tension/fatigue syndrome	Persistent lethargy
Kidney/bladder	Nephritis	Facial or ankle swelling/fluid retention
	Enuresis	'Wetting', discomfort with urination
Gastro-intestinal system	Mouth ulceration	Ulcers in mouth
	Enteropathy	Abdominal pain/distension

Condition	Symptom(s)
Colitis	Diarrhoea
Proctitis	Inflammation of lower bowel
Musculo-skeletal system Arthritis	Painful, swollen joints
Arthralgia	Aching joints and limbs

Before we look at these in detail, it is as well to have a working knowledge of the language and basic facts involved in allergy. You will then have a clear understanding of the principles of allergy management:

- The tendency towards allergy is an inherited trait.
- If one parent has an allergy, then the chances of one or more of the children developing an allergy are doubled.
- If both parents are allergic, then the risk for their children increases fourfold.
- Specific allergic conditions are not necessarily inherited. This means that a father with asthma may not necessarily have a child with the same complaint. That child might develop eczema or hay fever, or even be totally free of allergies.
- An atopic child is one who has an inherited tendency to develop allergies.
- An allergen is a substance capable of producing an allergic reaction, e.g. grass pollen when it causes asthma.
- An allergic reaction is an abnormal response to a substance that is tolerated well by normal (that is, non-allergic) individuals. The reaction can occur to allergens which are inhaled, consumed in food or drink, injected, or which come into contact with the skin.

Here are some examples:

Allergen	Allergic reaction
House dust (inhaled)	Asthma
Eggs (consumed)	Eczema
Nickel (contact)	Dermatitis
Penicillin (injected)	Urticaria

THE ALLERGIC CONDITIONS OF CHILDHOOD

The three classic allergies are asthma, eczema and hay fever. The most common inhaled allergens are: house-dust mites (insects which live in household dust), house dust, animal danders, grass pollen, tree pollen, weed/shrub pollens and moulds. And the most common foodstuffs capable of causing allergies include: milk, fish, wheat, eggs and peanuts.

The list is, in fact, quite extensive. In the case of some children many different foods are involved in their illnesses, while others may be sensitive only to one or two food groups.

Some atopic children go through the full range of allergic reactions quite early on in life. Michael developed problems at the age of eight months. His father was a hay-fever sufferer and his mother had had asthma as a child. This immediately increased his chances of developing one of the major allergies, which eventually presented as eczema. His mother noticed that certain foods – especially eggs – made the eczema worse and kept them out of his diet. Also, his skin improved considerably when she took him off milk formula.

Michael seemed to be only just growing out of eczema when asthma set in. This followed a stay in a rather dusty holiday home, and his parents noticed how sensitive to dust he became after that. The asthma was soon controlled by the use of medication, but a year later, during the summer months, he developed what was quite obviously hay fever.

Michael, for some unknown reason, had gone through all three of the classic allergies within his first five years of life! His allergic nature had responded to allergens consumed and inhaled. It is these two main areas of response that cause most childhood allergies, and we shall concentrate on them throughout the book.

2

Allergies of the Eyes, Ears, Nose and Chest

Coughs, wheezes, runny noses, and earaches represent a major part of the general practice work-load in every country. Parents of young children know only too well how often they attend their family doctors with these problems. They often leave the surgery armed with (yet another) prescription for an antibiotic, cough mixture or decongestant. These may make little impression on the symptoms, and some children appear to go from one course of an antibiotic straight on to another – and another, and another. Many of these children have an underlying allergic condition, and the symptoms are being wrongly diagnosed as due to infection.

We shall now discuss the features of allergy as it affects the eyes, ears, noses, sinuses and chests of children. Remember that the term 'allergen' means any substance capable of producing an allergic reaction (for instance, grass pollen as a cause of asthma). The medical terms used when describing these conditions usually end in '-itis', as in 'bronchitis' and 'sinusitis'. The '-itis' implies inflammation, and inflammation, broadly speaking, is caused either by infection or by allergy. The distinction between the two is important, as the treatment routines are very different.

Eye allergies – conjunctivitis

The conjunctiva is the white part of the eye, and in conjunctivitis this becomes red and itchy. The redness is caused by a marked increase in and swelling of the small blood vessels which are on the conjunctiva. Children with allergic conjunctivitis look as if they have been 'out on the town' a lot! In addition to the redness and itch there is an excessive amount of watering and repeated blinking. The lower eyelids become thickened by the rubbing to relieve the constant itch.

8

These symptoms can occur on an all-year-round or seasonal-only basis (usually the summer months). Occasionally a child will have the all-year-round features with a worsening during the summer. This reflects the particular allergen that is causing the problem. All-year-round symptoms are usually due to house-dust mites. Summer-only features are usually due to grass, tree pollen. Symptoms occurring all year round but worse in summer are usually due to dust mites, pollens.

The summer-only form of conjunctivitis can produce rather dramatic-looking symptoms: the white part of the eye swells and looks like jelly. There is considerable redness, watering and some blurring of vision.

The combination of allergic conjunctivitis and allergic rhinitis (see below) occurring during the summer months is popularly known as hay fever. This really is a misnomer, as the condition is not caused by hay and does not produce a fever.

Nasal allergies – rhinitis

'Blow your nose properly', 'Stop sniffing' – how many times have you heard these commands from the mothers of young children? Runny-nosed kids are so common that it hardly seems necessary to pay special attention to their problem. Yet the fact is that many of them have to keep sniffing because of the itch and the mucus which are forever irritating their noses. They would like to blow their noses properly, as they have a constant feeling of pressure there – but they never seem to be able to clear them.

The principal features of allergic rhinitis are itch, sneezing, blockage and a clear mucus discharge. If the blockage is severe, the child will have a 'dropped chin' appearance. This occurs as the effort of breathing through the nose becomes too great and the chin is thus permanently dropped to allow mouth breathing. There may be a 'flat-faced' feature, where the normal folds of the cheeks at the side of the nose (naso-labial folds) are lost. A close look at the bridge of the nose may reveal a crease where the child has rubbed the nose upwards with the flat of the hand in order to gain relief from the itch.

Children with a nasal blockage tend to snore (or at least to have noisy breathing) when asleep. These symptoms are sometimes mistakenly thought to be due to enlarged adenoids, which are then surgically removed. Such an operation, however, produces little relief if the blockage inside the nose is left untreated.

The lining of the nose is soft and quite sensitive. Along the inside of it are 'shelves', called turbinates. Both the lining and the turbinates respond to various allergens by swelling. As they swell there is a mucus discharge – producing the runny nose – and a blockage of the nasal passage.

A further complication in this area is the formation of a nasal polyp. This is like a small grape and is the end product of a prolonged swelling of the lining of the nose and sinuses. When a polyp forms inside the nose there is an almost total blockage on the affected side and a feeling of permanent congestion. This is most uncomfortable. Fortunately, only about one per cent of allergic children develop polyps. Youngsters with asthma, eczema and nasal polyps must take care with their diet (see the section of this chapter on management, p. 15).

Like allergic conjunctivitis, rhinitis may be either a seasonal or an all-year-round problem. Unlike conjunctivitis, however, which is almost exclusively due to airborne allergens, allergic rhinitis may have a dietary cause.

Seasonal rhinitis occurs in the summer months when grass and/or tree pollens are in the air. Sneezing is more of a problem for seasonal sufferers than it is for those with the all-year-round variety. The nasal discharge is profuse and clear.

All-year-round rhinitis (whether or not there is a seasonal worsening of symptoms) may be caused exclusively by household allergens such as dust, feathers, etc., or a food allergy. The commonest food incriminated is cow's milk. Some children have both inhaled and food allergies, so attention must be paid to identifying both before relief can be obtained.

In addition to the nasal mucus associated with allergic rhinitis, some children also get 'post-nasal drip' or catarrh. This happens when mucus trickles down the back of the throat causing a repeated clearing of the throat. Some children prefer to keep swallowing the mucus: this will cause them no harm. Post-nasal drip or catarrh is notoriously difficult to treat, but it may respond to a diet that is free of dairy products.

Sinus allergies – sinusitis

The sinuses are air pockets in the bones of the skull which have an opening into the inside of the nose. They are lined with tissue which responds to allergens by swelling and secreting mucus.

Sinusitis, when allergic in nature, produces symptoms of pressure and congestion. The sufferer may complain of headaches, and at times there may be puffiness around the cheek-bones.

Seasonal conjunctivitis and rhinitis – hay fever

The collection of features that include red, itchy and watering eyes and an itchy, blocked and runny nose (with or without chest symptoms) is widely known as hay fever. Occasionally, too, there is an intense itch along the roof of the mouth and inside the ears. For years hay fever was regarded as nothing more than a nuisance, but coming as it does at the point of major school examinations it cannot be treated lightly. In addition to the physical symptoms affecting the nose and eyes and mentioned above, many children with hay fever become irritable and lethargic and tire easily. Until recently the types of treatment used actually caused a worsening of these symptoms: it was a toss-up which caused the worst problem, hay fever or its treatment! Fortunately there are new preparations available which give excellent results.

Quite often hay fever is accompanied by a persistent cough which is allergic bronchitis. Because the child may have runny eyes and nose and a cough the features may be mistaken for a head and chest 'cold'. Indeed, the two conditions look remarkably similar. A useful point to check is whether your child has an itchy nose or eyes. An itch points to an allergic rather than an infective cause.

Sixteen-year-old David was a hay-fever sufferer for many years, although the symptoms were only correctly interpreted when he was fourteen. Before that he was treated for summer 'colds' which lasted from March to September! One year his mother counted the number of different decongestants she had bought or been prescribed, and the total was twenty-four.

David disliked the summer months intensely: he always felt tired, lethargic and 'bunged up'. At this time, while most of his friends took advantage of the long, warm days to play sport, David found that his chest became very congested when he ran around, leaving him quite breathless. He avoided games as much as he could in the summer, which surprised everyone because in the winter months he was rarely off the playing fields.

In the long, hot summer of 1982 his hay fever became much worse: he was breathless with wheezing, constantly rubbing his itchy eyes and blowing his nose. While the high pollen count that summer brought on David's worst-ever attacks of hay fever, it at least made his doctor rethink the diagnosis. With the emphasis no longer on infection and now turned towards allergy, David improved dramatically.

Nowadays he has the appropriate preventive treatment at the end of spring and is free of hay fever in the summer. The change in his personality and physical drive is also for the better. As mid-June is the usual time for major examinations (and also for high pollen levels), the correct treatment at this point means David can approach any test in peak form.

Management

The management of such problems should be as follows: 1 specific treatment, 2 antihistamines, 3 cortisone preparations, 4 allergy testing and follow-up, and 5 desensitization.

ALLERGIES OF THE EYES, EARS, NOSE AND CHEST

Allergic conjunctivitis

1 *Specific treatment.* The most effective eye-drops used in allergic conjunctivitis are Opticrom and cortisone. Opticrom is extremely safe and very effective, whereas cortisone drops must be used with care and are probably better left until an eye specialist has checked the situation. They can be used over a short period for quick relief, after which Opticrom can be used. Opticrom drops are useful in treating both all-year-round and seasonal conjunctivitis.

2 *Antihistamines.* Antihistamines are not terribly effective in allergic conjunctivitis; certainly they do not bring the total relief that can be achieved with eye-drops. The newer antihistamines – Triludan and Hismanal – are the best for this condition.

3 *Cortisone preparations.* Cortisone can be given in the form of a tablet or an injection (as well as in the form of eye-drops). Used in short, sharp dosages they are quite safe, but long-term use in children is not recommended because of the side-effects. There is no reason for using long-term cortisone in allergic conjunctivitis. An injection form of cortisone called Kenalog or Depo-Medrone is quite popular as it lasts for up to six weeks. This method does away with the need for regular eye-drops, tablets, etc. and is quite useful in the treatment of seasonal conjunctivitis, particularly in children doing school exams. It is better not to have this more than twice in the season.

4 *Allergy testing and follow-up.* Allergy testing will confirm whether the problem is allergic in nature and identifies the responsible allergens. This is of more use in all-year-round conjunctivitis. If house-dust mites and dust, etc. are responsible for the symptoms, then appropriate anti-dust measures (see Chapter 7) may reduce the symptoms considerably and permit the tailing-off of treatment.

5 *Desensitization routines.* These are discussed in detail in Chapter 7.

Allergic rhinitis and sinusitis

1 *Specific treatments (nasal sprays).* Nasal sprays come in the form of two kinds of preparation: treatment and preventive. The most effective treatment sprays contain a form of cortisone. These are safe, very effective, and free of side-effects. They do not damage the lining of the nose with repeated use, nor do they interfere with natural cortisone production.

Preventive sprays are best used before symptoms come on – this is particularly true of seasonal rhinitis. However, they can be used for and are effective in the treatment of all-year-round rhinitis.

2 *Antihistamines.* Antihistamines are best used before symptoms appear – this is particularly true of seasonal rhinitis. The newer preparations of Triludan and Hismanal are relatively free of side-effects and can be administered to children. The best results seem to be obtained when one of the nasal sprays is used in combination with the antihistamines. Again, this is mainly of use in treating seasonal rhinitis.

3 *Cortisone preparations.* The other cortisone preparations come in the forms of tablets and injections. Tablets can be used in short, sharp dosages to gain maximum relief and then tailored off. They should not be used over long periods for children with allergic rhinitis. Injection preparations are usually of the long-acting variety which last up to six weeks. These are useful in seasonal rhinitis but should not be given more than twice in one summer.

4 *Allergy testing and follow-up.* Allergy tests confirm which allergens are responsible for the symptoms, allowing for a more comprehensive approach to management and a possible reduction in the amount of medication that is necessary. While household dusts, feathers, etc. are significant factors in all-year-round rhinitis, certain foods (particularly cow's milk) may also be involved. These may show on allergy testing, but more often

the suspicion is raised by the history of infant-feeding patterns and current symptoms. (This is discussed in more detail in Chapter 7.)

5 *Desensitization routines.* These are dealt with in Chapter 7.

The sinusitis will respond to the same routine as is used in rhinitis. Indeed, the sinus allergies will not clear if the nasal allergy is overlooked.

If there are nasal polyps present, then the only useful medications used for control are the cortisone nasal sprays. Should the child in question also suffer from asthma and eczema, then a dietary avoidance of azo-dyes and benzoate preservatives is important (see Chapter 8) as these may well aggravate all three conditions.

I have found the most effective treatments for hay fever to be either Triludan or Hismanal combined with one of the cortisone nasal sprays and Opticrom eye-drops; or, alternatively, for those children who tend to forget their medication or to get fed up with the routine, an injection of one of the long-acting cortisone preparations.

Do not treat hay fever lightly, as it definitely impairs physical and mental performance. This can mean the difference between good and bad grades at examination time for some children.

Allergies of the ear – serous otitis

In every child there is a short narrow-bore tube which connects the inner ear (that part behind the eardrum) to the back of the throat. This tube has three functions, namely ventilation of the inner ear, clearance of secretions produced in the inner ear, and protection of the inner ear from throat secretions.

In some allergic children the tube becomes blocked leading to an accumulation of secretions in the inner ear. Older children with this problem (known as serous otitis media) may complain of itchy, popping or stuffed-up ears. Some are not able to hear clearly and may appear disobedient by seeming to ignore requests made to them by those out of their range of vision. Younger children, as a rule, do not complain of anything, but they may have delayed language development because of hearing impairment.

Chronic serous otitis media may respond to an allergic approach. Identification of the allergens involved followed by removal or desensitization is one method of treatment. However, more often than not children suffering from this disorder end up having the fluid drained under anaesthetic and small tubes (grommets) inserted in the eardrum to prevent the reaccumulation of secretions.

Allergies of the eye, nose and ear – conclusion

Perhaps the most logical and successful approach to the above conditions is one that combines treatment, allergy evaluation and possible desensitization. If we consider the type of management used for David, it will become clear how this combined approach works.

David's hay fever was causing a great deal of problems and might well have interfered with his performance in public examinations had it been left unchecked. To bring him immediate relief from the symptoms he was put on a short (five-day) course of cortisone in tablet form. This cleared up the hay fever quite quickly. On the fourth day of treatment he started using eye-drops, a nasal spray and one of the new antihistamines (Hismanal). This treatment kept the symptoms at bay when the short course of cortisone was complete and allowed him to follow a normal life-style for the rest of the summer.

Later in the year he was skin-tested to confirm which pollens were causing his symptoms, and a desensitization schedule began before the following spring. This continued for three consecutive years, lasting ten weeks on each occasion. This meant that David had an injection each week from the beginning of January with the course being completed by mid-March. This desensitization procedure 'damped down' his body's reponse to pollen and allowed him to reduce significantly the amount of medication he needed for total relief. Nowadays he uses an antihistamine only during the very high pollen days in summer and is free from hay fever for the rest of the time.

This 'combination' approach to management is the most successful I have found and one I would recommend. To rely on drug treatment alone without identifying and trying an anti-allergy programme is illogical. Equally wrong is an over-emphasis on allergy management at the expense of using the safe, effective drug treatments. This really only prolongs the symptoms unnecessarily.

Allergies of the chest – asthma

This is a most significant problem in children, and is definitely on the increase. As many as ten per cent of all youngsters suffer from asthma, and while not all of them are allergic a considerable proportion do respond to anti-allergy measures.

The word 'asthma' means 'difficulty in breathing', and it occurs when the small tubes which carry air in and out of the lungs become narrowed and/or inflamed. This is accompanied by a number of symptoms, ranging from a persistent cough to wheezing and shortness of breath.

The features of asthma

Occasionally, in discussions with parents on the various features of asthma, they are surprised to learn that an important early symptom is a cough. This is particularly true if the cough is of a persistent or recurring nature. In many cases the child will cough only at night.

This is possibly one of the major stumbling-blocks experienced by doctors in dealing with some families: to such parents, the idea that a simple cough can mean asthma seems ridiculous. They tend to think of asthmatic children as being forever wheezing, too ill to play and sometimes being carted off to hospital in the middle of the night with distressed breathing. One or other parent may say: 'Doctor, is it not just a simple chest infection? Wouldn't an antibiotic clear everything up?' In fact, if it were just an infection, then an antibiotic would indeed do the trick. Yet in the case of a substantial proportion of children with repeated 'chest problems', infection plays merely a minor role.

Let us look at a simple but graphic example of this. Ann and Claire are identical twins and as alike as peas in a pod; it is almost impossible to tell them apart. However, for a few years there were certain features of Ann's general state of health which marked her out as very different from her sister.

Their father, John, explained it like this: 'Ann had a rather gaunt look about her which was very distinct compared to Claire. For months on end she seemed to need an antibiotic for her chest. Every cold settled on her chest. She was lighter than Claire, and not as active.'

Ann's mother, Terri, remembers her having repeated nights of coughing which usually ended in a vomiting episode. 'Ann's chest problem meant that she missed quite a lot of school and kept her from being as active as her twin. She couldn't keep up with Claire when they played together,' she recalls. Terri felt that Ann looked tense and apprehensive during these periods of ill health.

Ann is now totally on top of her chest problem – which turned out to be asthma – and can actually outrun Claire nowadays. She is relaxed, more active and generally better all round. Her recovery dates from when anti-asthma medication was introduced. Because the traditionally recognized features of asthma – wheezing and shortness of breath – were not prominent in Ann's case, the diagnosis may have been delayed.

Coughs, wheezes and shortness of breath

We saw in Ann's story that a persistent cough was the main symptom. Yet at times she also wheezed and got short of breath.

Next to a cough, wheezing is the second main feature of asthma. A wheeze can be described as a musical sound – sometimes like a whistle, occasionally like the sound of an organ – coming from the chest. It may be brought on only by exercise, or by a head cold, or in dusty surroundings. Alternatively, the sufferer may wheeze all the time.

If your child wheezes, he or she will almost certainly have some degree of breathlessness, however mild. This may, again, only become noticeable with exercise or if the wheeze becomes pronounced.

Wrong labels

It is now considered that the following diagnostic labels no longer mean anything in themselves and usually mask an underlying asthma: recurrent bronchitis, wheezy bronchitis, 'bronchial', 'chestiness' and allergic cough.

Variations on these terms may well occur in different parts of the country, but these are the most frequently used. Some doctors are also suspicious about the casual way in which whooping cough is given as a diagnosis in some cases. Quite often this occurs when a persistent cough defies the traditional treatments of cough mixtures and antibiotics.

Over-sensitive airways and subtle asthma

Some children have what can only be adequately described as over-sensitive airways (lung tubes): on receiving even slight stimuli, the airways react by narrowing. These children usually cough during such events. Occasionally the cough may sound indistinguishable from croup, which has a seal-like 'barking' quality.

The stimuli which trigger such reactions include cold air, exercise and smoky atmospheres. Not every child with over-sensitive airways goes on to develop asthma, though a proportion do so. Croup may well be a variation of the 'over-sensitive airways' condition. Persistent or recurring 'over-sensitive airways' symptoms can be either reversed or prevented with the use of an appropriate anti-asthma medication.

Subtle asthma affects children without them displaying any of the classical features of asthma proper, such as coughing or wheezing. Not infrequently such children are the brothers or sisters of a diagnosed asthmatic child. The features include excessive perspiration and an unusually red face on taking exercise. Some children just seem to be always under par or unduly tired on a regular basis; they are difficult to spot unless the problem is specifically sought for. This form of asthma is so subtle that the child's symptoms are usually vague and ill-defined. I would describe such children as having an invisible ball and chain around the leg. They just seem unable to perform many tasks with maximum effort. Such patients respond excellently to anti-asthma treatment and very soon lose this trait.

A question score card for diagnosis

We now have sufficient information to devise a scoring system for identifying asthma in children. Put the following questions to yourself, and add up the score at the end. For every 'yes', award two points. There are no points for a 'no' answer.

		Yes	No
A	*Cough symptoms*		
1	Does your child have a persistent or recurring cough?		
2	Does your child cough when making physical effort?		
3	Does your child cough a lot at night?		
B	*Wheeze and shortness of breath*		
4	Does your child wheeze a lot?		
5	Does your child wheeze or get unduly short of breath with physical exercise?		
6	Does your child wheeze with every head cold?		
C	*Wrong labels*		
7	Does your child have 'recurring bronchitis', 'wheezy bronchitis'?		
8	Does your child miss a lot of school because of chest problems?		
9	Has your child been described as 'bronchial'?		

Yes   *No*

D   *Family history*

10   Is there a family history of asthma, eczema, hay fever?

11   Is there a family history of croup, bronchitis?

12   Has your child ever had eczema?

Score:

2–6: Very suggestive of asthma

6 and over: Definite asthma

There are other causes of cough, wheeze and shortness of breath in children. However, for all practical purposes the above question score card will identify accurately the majority of asthma sufferers.

Let us look at a practical use of the scoring system as used in the case of a particular child. Sandra – aged six – has had chest problems on and off for two years. Her usual treatment routine involved an antibiotic plus a cough mixture. These made little impression, and she remained below par for most of this time.

Sandra's mother answered 'yes' to questions 1, 2, 3, 5, 6, 7 and 8, giving her a total of fourteen points – well above the lowest score for asthma diagnosis. Physical examination confirmed that Sandra had asthma, and she was put on appropriate treatment. Her symptoms cleared totally within one week, and she remained free from all symptoms for some months while on a preventive treatment routine. After about four months' continual therapy she stopped all medication and has remained asthma-free to this day.

The causes of asthma

The commonest causes of asthma in children include infections, environmental pollution, emotion, exertion and allergies. Let us consider each in detail.

Infections. These are caused either by viruses or by bacteria. Viruses cause such common illnesses as influenza and measles, while bacteria cause bronchitis, meningitis, etc.

Because small children have to develop their own immunity to infections, in other words build up an adequate defence system to prevent their recurrence, they tend to develop viral infections more readily than do adults. A child with a tendency towards asthma who gets a head cold may well end up coughing and wheezing. If the cough or wheeze persists for long enough, bacteria may come along as 'secondary invaders' and settle in the inflamed lungs, causing a true chest infection. This will almost certainly make the asthma worse as well.

As a general rule, bacteria do not cause asthma: rather, they cause an infection in addition to the asthma. The bacterial 'bugs' are caught in the inflamed lung tubes – like flies on flypaper – and multiply there.

Environmental pollution. By this I mean cigarette smoke, car exhaust fumes, industrial and household smog. The most significant one here is cigarette smoke. If you have an asthmatic child you would be quite wrong to smoke in the same room as him or her.

Emotion. For the vast majority of asthmatic children emotional upsets play no part in their illness. However, having asthma which is not properly controlled can cause these children to suffer from problems of an emotional nature. It is fascinating to learn of youngsters previously described as irritable, cranky and temperamental, whose personalities improve considerably when their asthma is brought under proper control.

Exertion. Some children will only cough, wheeze or become short of breath on taking exercise. An important distinction should be made here between the child with incompletely controlled asthma made worse by physical exertion and the one with true 'exercise-induced' asthma. The former may only require a change in medication for the control of symptoms brought on by physical exertion. The 'exercise-induced' asthmatic, on the other hand, is well and free of symptoms except when running or taking some other form of vigorous exercise. The asthma may come on suddenly or may be delayed for some minutes. Children who have 'late exercise' asthma will be fine at sprinting but not so good at middle-distance or long runs.

Allergies. The allergies which cause asthma are either inhaled or consumed in food or drink, and the majority of asthmatic children can be shown to have an allergic tendency. How important this is in the condition is not completely clear, and certainly any approach that is based purely on allergic lines and omits to treat the symptoms is unlikely to succeed.

Allergy tests will identify accurately the substances to which the child is allergic. These tests are useful in the case of such allergens as dusts, moulds, pollens, etc., but they are not so reliable when it comes to foods.

Let us consider the commonest inhaled allergens and discuss ways of dealing with them. On testing, positive results are usually shown to house-dust mites, house dust, feathers, animal danders, moulds and pollens. This suggests that such substances, when inhaled, can cause or aggravate asthma. The management format, which is based on the results of allergy testing, is best explained by looking at individual cases.

Peter, aged nine, has wheezed for most of his life. In infancy he had eczema and colic and was described as an irritable baby. During the summer months he suffers from what is very obviously hay fever.

Allergy testing shows Peter to be allergic to dust mites, dust, feathers, pollens and cow's milk. In a two-stage treatment his bedroom was made as dust-free as possible (see Chapter 7) and his pillows and duvet changed to others made from a non-allergenic material. This greatly alleviated his chest condition and also the associated allergies of rhinitis and conjunctivitis. Yet his wheezing did not disappear completely. In the second stage of treatment he was put on a milk-free diet for six weeks. His asthma almost completely cleared after a week, and his parents noticed how much less medication was required to keep him well.

As we have seen, this child's problems were caused by both inhaled and consumed allergic reactions, both of which required attention before control was achieved.

It is considered that no more than ten per cent of childhood asthma is due to a food allergy. However, for these children dietary manipulation can lead to an improvement in their condition. The foods most frequently found to cause problems are cow's milk, cheese, eggs, wheat, yeast, fish, pork and peanuts. The artificial colourings and preservatives used in many of today's foodstuffs can also provoke asthma in children who are susceptible. For some unknown reason, Asian children can develop episodes of wheezing in response to eating crisps, chips, coloured sweets and ice cream.

Points to look for which suggest a food allergy association in asthma include a history of eczema, feeding difficulties in infancy, a finicky appetite, irritability, poor sleep and difficulty in concentration. The combination of asthma, eczema and nasal polyps increases the likelihood of a sensitivity to salicylates (see Chapter 8). These are present in aspirin and aspirin-containing medicines. Indeed, many across-the-counter cough mixtures contain aspirin and should be avoided. Quite often, salicylate-sensitive children also react to azo-dyes and benzoate food preservatives. If your child has asthma and eczema (with or without nasal polyps) it is probably better to use paracetamol only as an analgesic.

The treatment of childhood asthma

There are three stages of change in the lungs of children with asthma. Each stage causes further breathing problems and must be reversed before total control can be achieved.

The asthma sequence is as follows:

Normal air tube $\longrightarrow$ (bronchus)

Stage 1: Narrowed air tube due to muscle contraction (bronchoconstriction)

↓

Stage 2: Further narrowing due to combination of muscle contraction and swelling of the inner lining of the lung tube

↓

Stage 3: As Stages 1 and 2, with the addition of mucus production and secretion into air tube

In many children, the only event to occur is Stage 1, and this may revert either spontaneously or with treatment.

The changes take place in the tiny tubes which carry air in and out of the lungs. Each tube is surrounded by muscle tissue and lined with a sensitive layer of tissue. In asthma the outer muscle layer contracts, causing the tube to narrow. Not long afterwards the tube's inner lining starts to swell and secretes mucus (or phlegm). Consequently the lung tubes are narrowed by the swollen inner lining and the outer muscle contraction.

Drugs are available which are capable of reversing all three stages of the asthma sequence (see Appendix 3). There is also a preventive drug which can be used to keep asthma at bay once control has been achieved. The choice of drug preparation is very much an individual decision on the part of the doctor. However, the inhaled forms are safe, quick and most effective. The tablet and syrup forms have the disadvantages of being slower in action, associated with side-effects and likely to contain troublesome colouring agents.

Stage 1 drugs (bronchodilators). These reverse the muscle contraction and can be given by injection, orally in tablet or syrup form, by inhalation or by suppository. The suppository form is messy, inconvenient and unpredictable. (A list of Stage 1 drugs is given in Appendix 3.)

Stages 2 and 3 drugs (cortisone preparations). Cortisone is extremely useful when the asthma sequence has gone past Stage 1 as it will reverse the swelling of the tube lining and 'dry up' the production of mucus. It is available in tablet and injection form; there are also aerosol inhaler and rotacap variations of the same drug. The long-term use of tablet or injection forms of cortisone is associated with quite troublesome side-effects. The aerosol inhaler and rotacap preparations do not cause such problems when the recommended dosage is used.

Generally speaking, the Stage 2 cortisone preparations are introduced when Stage 1 drugs fail to control asthma symptoms completely; this suggests that the asthma sequence has progressed to either Stage 2 or Stage 3. Almost as soon as one is added there is complete relief of symptoms and, in the case of some children, their first asthma-free days for months.

The tablet and injection forms of cortisone are reserved for asthma attacks or severe asthma that does not respond to inhaled cortisone. This is quite rare.

Occasionally, if a child is very 'mucusy' and distressed with wheezing, the inhaled sprays will fail to penetrate deeply enough into the lungs to achieve their effect. In these situations a short course of cortisone given by tablet or injection will 'dry up' the lungs, allowing the sprays to penetrate better. In the case of these short, sharp dosages there are no side-effects. (A list of Stage 2 drugs is given in Appendix 3.)

Preventive drugs (Intal and steroid inhalers). After an asthmatic child has been treated and if there are no further symptoms, it is useful to remove the treatment drugs and introduce a preventive medication. One preparation that is commonly used in this situation is Intal (sodium cromoglycate). This rather unique drug appears to work by stabilizing the lung tubes and preventing the asthma sequence from recurring. It is particularly useful in children. While it is more logical to use Intal when the asthma sequence has been reversed completely, it is quite often used earlier to good effect.

Intal is a medication that is completely safe and free of side-effects. It is available in the forms of an aerosol inhaler, a spincap and a respirator solution. While Intal does not work for every asthmatic child, it is worth a trial as the results are exellent and the medication is so safe. If Intal is introduced early enough into the treatment routine of an asthmatic child, it may be unnecessary to use Stage 2 and 3 drugs.

For those sufferers who fail to respond to Intal, the steroid inhalers – Becotide, Pulmicort, Bextasol and Becloforte – can also be used as preventives.

Asthma – conclusion

The treatment of childhood asthma with medication involves reversing each of the stages of the asthma sequence in a step-by-step fashion. When the lung tubes are restored to their non-asthmatic state it is worth while introducing a preventive medication to prevent a recurrence of symptoms.

Problems

The only problems that might occur with these treatments tend to arise after control has been achieved: because the patient seems so well, both parents and children forget about the need to keep a close eye on the situation.

When a breakdown in treatment occurs, it is generally due to one of the following:

1 Inhaler routines being rushed and poorly performed.
2 Inhaler techniques being forgotten and incorrectly performed.
3 Dosage and frequency of medication being forgotten.
4 Parents/child getting fed up with the routine and neglecting to carry it through.
5 Treatments being stopped too soon as the results are so good (asthma tends to return quite quickly in this situation).
6 A well-meaning friend or relative saying, 'That's too strong/not good/useless for your child. My brother/sister/cousin was on that, and it did him/her no good.'

There are many variations on this kind of misguided advice, but do remember that asthma has such an individual effect on children that not every child will find the same treatment useful.

Should you have any worries or fears about your child's treatment, discuss them with your doctor or specialist. Don't lightly discard their advice on the strength of careless suggestions from outsiders.

Other kinds of drug treatment

Some doctors use two other drug groups in treating asthma: Zaditen and antihistamines. Zaditen stabilizes the cells in the lung tubes, which seem to be unusually fragile in asthma. Unfortunately it is not a very effective drug, although some asthmatic children may find it useful.

Antihistamines are generally of no use in asthma, except when dealing with the true pollen-only form. Even then they are not as effective as the other types of medication discussed.

3

Allergies Affecting the Brain

These are migraine, epilepsy, hyperactivity and the tension/fatigue syndrome. Evidence is mounting that certain foods can cause a wide range of symptoms related to brain activity. What is not completely certain is whether the foods cause a true allergic reaction or whether the response is a peculiarity of the individual concerned. Some doctors believe that the reactions may be due to a pharmacological action of the constituents of foodstuffs; in simple terms, this means that they act like a drug.

It is probably better to describe the symptoms brought on by consuming various foodstuffs as caused by food intolerance rather than by food allergy. In practical terms, the treatment is the same: avoid the offending food.

Migraine

This is a condition – afflicting adults and children alike – whose main feature is a persistent or recurring headache. Nausea and vomiting may also take place. Some sufferers experience bright, flashing lights or feelings of intense hunger before an attack of migraine.

In children, the main feature is headache. The child may be irritable or bad-tempered and want to lie down. He or she will have a furrowed brow during these episodes, and may complain of feeling sick. Migraine in children occurs in about five per cent of boys and girls by the age of eleven, and there is often a family history of the problem.

It is most important that the headaches are assessed by a doctor to ensure that no other causes are involved.

In children whose migraine is known to be caused by foodstuffs there may well be other, associated problems. If your child has migraine plus one or more of the following symptoms, then food intolerance should be suspected:

29

Stomach pains	Runny nose
Diarrhoea	Recurring mouth ulcers
Flatulence	Asthma
Overactivity	Eczema
Aching limbs	Vaginal discharge

The foodstuffs that are most frequently incriminated are: cow's milk, eggs, chocolate, oranges, wheat, benzoic acid (a food additive), cheese, tomatoes and tartrazine (a food additive).

In fact quite a range of different foods are involved in this problem, and for some children the headaches may be caused by eating several different ones.

If your child suffers from food-related migraine and the complaint is managed accordingly, then other events which might in the past have provoked a headache may no longer have the same effect. These include such things as exercise, bright lights, noise, extremes of temperature and bangs on the head.

Epilepsy

There are different forms of this condition, ranging from convulsions or *grand mal* to *petit mal*, in which the child 'turns off' and becomes oblivious to his or her surroundings. Some children have convulsive episodes with high temperatures.

Recent research has shown that certain foods can provoke both high temperatures and convulsions in those children who are susceptible. In cases where food is definitely a factor, putting the child on a diet free of the problem foods can relieve the condition. Indeed, such patients can also be taken off their anti-epileptic medication.

As with migraine, the children who have other allergic features (asthma, rhinitis, eczema, etc.) tend to respond better to dietary treatment. In particular, those children with histories of fever-induced convulsions or recurring, unexplained fevers are more likely to respond to a dietary approach. The doctors who investigated the food–epilepsy connection also noted that the boy:girl ratio was three to one, with a preponderance of blond-haired, blue-eyed boys.

The foodstuffs most frequently found to cause symptoms in this condition are: cow's milk, cheese, citrus fruits and chocolate.

Hyperactivity

This is a controversial and poorly defined condition of children, with features as set out below. It appears to be more common in boys than in girls, and is not always associated with an allergic nature. The role of foodstuffs in provoking symptoms is now accepted, and treatment by dietary methods is quite often successful.

At his or her most extreme, the hyperactive child is an absolute monster beyond the control of parents, teachers or doctors. There would appear to be a wide variation in the symptoms of hyperactivity, and some sufferers show only mild features. One of the main difficulties lies in deciding whether the child in question really is hyperactive in the true, medical sense of the word or is just behaving in a way that is normal but somewhat over-exuberant. Occasionally, parents who are ill-equipped to deal with their offspring use the label 'hyperactive' as a shield to hide behind, when their child's behaviour is actually a reflection of their own inadequacies.

Thomas, aged six, was taken to the doctor by his parents, who wanted advice on how to deal with his 'over-activity'. It appeared that he was bold, aggressive, disobedient and constantly in trouble with his father. After a long and often heated discussion, it was revealed that Thomas's parents were on the point of splitting up. His father was a heavy drinker who often struck his wife and shouted at her in front of their child; on more than one occasion Thomas had tried to shield his mother from the physical abuse. When the child's teachers complained about his behaviour at school and suggested he was seen by a psychologist, his father decided that something had to be done. He had read of the 'hyperactive child' syndrome and felt sure that his son fitted the picture.

Few children will develop placid and tranquil personalities in such an environment, and Thomas was no exception. His behaviour was a response to his unhappy, violent home life. Indeed he improved only after his parents separated and he was in his mother's sole care.

Thomas's story is by no means unique, but what is interesting is the way in which his father tried to deflect attention and blame away from his problems on to the child with a contrived suggestion of hyperactivity.

The truly hyperactive child will show many of the following features:

Restlessness or over-activity
Excitability or impulsiveness
Disturbs other children
Short attention span
Constantly fidgeting
Easily distracted
Demands must be met immediately
Easily frustrated
Cries often and easily
Quick mood changes
Temper outbursts
Intense thirst

In addition there may be other features of food intolerance, such as headaches, tummy pains, a runny nose, aching limbs, eczema, asthma and mouth ulcers. The foodstuffs most frequently incriminated in this condition are: artificial colourings and preservatives, cow's milk, chocolate, grapes, wheat, oranges, cheese, eggs and peanuts.

As with the migraine–food relationship, some hyperactive children are affected by many different foods while others may be troubled by only a few. The occasional sufferer may have behavioural problems as a result of inhalant reactions to pollens, dusts and perfumes. With the majority of hyperactive children, however, foodstuffs are to blame.

One very interesting feature of hyperactivity is a marked thirst. This is a useful guide to management as most of the children are free of this symptom when on a correct diet. It is surprising how many highly allergic children have thirst among their symptoms, and no theory has yet been put forward to explain why this should occur.

Tension/fatigue syndrome

It is possible that some allergic children have a collection of ill-defined symptoms which keep them constantly below par. They are often described as being 'run-down'. The features here include:

Nervous tension
Fatigue
Anxiety
Difficulties with lessons

Sleeplessness
Headaches
Listlessness
A general appearance of ill health

They sometimes have dark rings under the eyes with puffiness of the surrounding skin, known as allergic shiners.

Whether these features are due to a specific problem, such as asthma or eczema, or really reflect a separate condition is difficult to say. However, many of the symptoms clear when the diet is modified.

Management

When considering each of the conditions discussed in this chapter it is important to remember that other illnesses can produce similar symptoms. For this reason it is essential to have your doctor assess the situation before any conclusions are drawn as to whether the problem is food-related or not. There are separate features to check for in the history of infant feeding which will provide clues as to food intolerance (see Chapter 7).

Identifying which foods are involved in these conditions can be quite difficult. Skin tests are occasionally helpful, but more often than not only an 'elimination and challenge' diet will pinpoint the exact culprits (see Chapter 7). It is most important that any diet is checked either by a doctor or a trained nutritionist before your child is treated in this way.

In treating the 'hyperactive' syndrome, dietary manipulation plus the use of evening primrose oil is very helpful. This is particularly so in the case of those children who have thirst as a feature of their condition. Evening primrose oil is an essential fatty acid rich in linoleic acid and gamma linoleic acid. It has proved to be an important dietary supplement in many conditions, including hyperactivity.

One of the most interesting and satisfactory results of treating children with food intolerance is the number of associated symptoms which clear up in addition to the original problem.

Peter was described by his parents and teachers as uncontrollable. He was markedly over-active, always on the go, constantly fidgeting and rarely able to concentrate on any one activity. He seemed to be always in trouble at school, and disrupted other children at playtime. In infancy he had had eczema, colic and constipation when weaned on to a cow's milk formula. He was described as a difficult, irritable baby. As he grew older he became 'chesty' with every head cold, was very active physically and was noticed to have an intense thirst. He consumed bottles of orange squash every day.

During a visit to the family doctor for a flare-up of Peter's chest trouble, his mother raised the possibility of his having allergy problems. The doctor listened to the list of symptoms and agreed with the allergy suggestion.

As an experiment, Peter was put on a milk-free, colouring- and preservative-free diet for one month. Within the first week he showed a remarkable improvement in temperament, behaviour and concentration. His thirst was still present, although not on such a dramatic scale. On one occasion he broke his diet by having a large glass of orange squash, and within hours he became irritable, moody and agitated and had a remarkably high colouring in his cheeks and ears. The orange squash contained one of the forbidden colouring agents which had been eliminated from his diet.

Further adjustments were made to the diet, which was then

supplemented with evening primrose oil. After three months of this routine, Peter's true personality shone through: he was a normal, well-adjusted child capable of joining in every school activity without disruption. What is more, his chest problems subsided, as did the almost ignored minor symptoms of aching limbs and headaches.

This diet did produce results, and has improved the quality of life all round for Peter and his family.

4

Allergies Affecting the Skin

In general terms, the three most important allergic reactions affecting the skin of children are urticaria, angio-oedema and atopic eczema.

Urticaria and angio-oedema

Urticaria is probably better known as 'hives', and looks like a blistering or wealing of the skin surface. The surrounding skin is red, as are the weals, and there is an intense itching. The weals can affect any area of the body, and usually last less than twenty-four hours.

Angio-oedema is really the same as urticaria, except that it affects the deeper skin layers. When there is generalized angio-oedema, the skin looks grossly swollen and the facial features can be distorted. We shall consider urticaria and angio-oedema together, as in many cases the causes are the same.

There are four distinct varieties of urticaria, namely: contact urticaria, physical urticaria, hereditary angio-oedema and 'ordinary' urticaria. The commonest of these is contact urticaria, which generally occurs as a result of contact with an allergenic substance. There is swelling, redness and itching, and the area involved will depend on where the allergen has touched the skin. For example, some children develop urticaria of the hands if they touch egg white, and should they lick their fingers the swelling or itch may erupt on their lips as well. The most frequently encountered allergens in respect of contact urticaria are foods and animal danders – especially those of cats, dogs and horses.

Physical urticaria implies that the weal/itch response is provoked by pressure on the skin surface. One form of this is known as dermographism, a condition in which it is possible to 'write' words on the skin and watch the weal rise up to form the individual letters. Another – rather sinister – form of physical urticaria can occur when the skin cools. This can be quite problematic as it quite often goes unrecognized and can lead to loss of consciousness during swimming, which can lead to drowning.

The majority of child sufferers fit into the 'ordinary' urticaria category, and here it is certain foods and drugs which are responsible. Only in a small number of cases is this type of urticaria related to underlying disease.

With foods, two distinctly different reactions are involved in producing urticaria: an immediate response and a late response. Foods which produce immediate urticaria include: eggs, milk, nuts, fish, shellfish, yeast and strawberries. The child may complain of tingling inside the mouth and have tummy pains after eating one of these substances. There will be large, intensely itchy weals on the face, body and limbs. Not infrequently the child will vomit, or later he or she will develop diarrhoea.

Because of the quick reaction involved here medical aid is frequently unnecessary: the parents merely observe the response and learn to avoid that food in the future. Occasionally even traces of the offending foods can give rise to problems, and details of these need to be noted for those occasions when the child is at parties and so on.

Urticaria lasting more than one month (chronic urticaria) requires a more careful evaluation: the foods and medicines the child takes need checking, and attention must be paid to whether the reaction occurs after contact with animals, chemicals, jewellery or clothing. Among foods, common offenders as far as chronic urticaria is concerned include seafood, nuts and eggs. Penicillin may be a causative agent, and the residues present in dairy products often complicate the picture. Aspirin (and aspirin-containing compounds), tartrazine dye and benzoate preservatives are recognized as being implicated in chronic urticaria (see Chapter 8).

One interesting – though confusing – problem occurs in relation to the coloured tablets used in treatment routines. If your child develops an urticarial reaction to, say, a penicillin tablet with a red coating, which has caused the reaction – the penicillin or the dye used in the coating? A simple method of deciding is to wash off the outer colouring and try the tablet again. In most cases the drug can then be tolerated. This is more than just an academic exercise, as it is not a good idea to have your child incorrectly labelled 'allergic to penicillin': this rules out a most important group of antibiotics that are useful in treating infectious illnesses.

The treatment of urticaria involves identifying the provocative allergens – usually by means of dietary elimination. In the case of chronic urticaria, one of the new antihistamines called Hismanal is effective in blocking the response.

An urticarial reaction to a food can sometimes be dramatic and involve an allergic response throughout the body. It might begin with, say, vomiting, abdominal pains and wheezing and lead on to swelling of the face, limbs and joints; there may also be intense itching. The condition looks alarming, and quite often calls for medical treatment. However, in many cases by the time the doctor has arrived the worst is over.

Atopic eczema

Of all the childhood allergies this condition is, I feel, the most distressing. It affects up to five per cent of all children, and the incidence is on the increase. It tends to be a condition of the very young, with most sufferers developing it before the end of their first year.

The events tend to occur in the following order. First, at around three or four months of age a patchy red irritating rash develops on the cheeks. Not long afterwards the rash worsens until the cheeks are raw and weeping. Then, when the child is about four to six months old the rash becomes established on the body, arms and legs, eventually settling in the creases of the elbows, wrists, buttocks, knees and ankles.

The hallmark of eczema is the intense itch, with the skin going through stages of redness, scaling, weeping and bleeding. The bleeding is brought on by scratching. The skin tends to be dry on the whole, and is particularly so on the scalp. Not every child with patchy eczema goes on to develop troublesome body eczema; indeed, sometimes only the facial area is affected. Some children with eczema show other associated allergic features such as asthma, rhinitis, conjunctivitis and multiple food intolerances.

Atopic eczema is a complex disorder involving allergic mechanisms of the intestine, skin and respiratory tract. These may produce an accumulative response the end-result of which is an inflammation of the skin.

It is felt that the allergic sequence begins in the intestines, where responses to certain foodstuffs trigger off the release of chemical agents which circulate in the bloodstream and deposit in the skin, producing inflammation. In addition, other allergens – notably, pollens and house-dust mites – entering through the respiratory tract also set off allergic reactions which will add to or exaggerate the initial problem. To add insult to injury, allergens coming into contact with inflamed skin cause allergic reactions on the skin surface which exacerbate the eczematous areas.

The foods thought to be involved in producing the initial skin inflammation are cow's milk and eggs, and the adoption of a diet from which these are excluded will often lead to an improvement in the condition.

If the eczema is quite troublesome, it may well be worth considering cutting out chicken and beef as well, since the proteins present in these are identical to those found in eggs and milk respectively. In addition, azo-dyes and benzoate preservatives (see Chapter 8) may aggravate eczema, though it is not certain whether this is an allergic mechanism or not.

The other allergens which are implicated in eczema include pollens, house-dust mites and animal danders. These may cause problems either by settling on inflamed skin or by entering the bloodstream via the respiratory tract.

The treatment of eczema involves attention to all three areas of possible allergic reaction: the intestine, the skin and the respiratory tract. The most important area for care here is the skin: many a child is denied relief from the appalling discomfort of eczema because of an over-reliance on dietary and other methods.

There is a very simple and effective 'step-ladder' approach to skin care involving the use of cortisone-based creams of varying strengths. These creams work by reducing the inflammation of the skin, and which used sensibly have no side-effects. Together with moisturizers, they are the mainstay of eczema treatment.

In essence, a strong cream is used initially to control the skin and achieve clearance of the eczema. A step-by-step reduction is then made in the strength of cream used (from strong through moderate to weak) until the eczema is seen to reappear. This is the 'cut-off' point for control. If we now go one step back up the ladder and use a slightly stronger cream, the 'breakthrough' eczema will clear. After a week, a further reduction is attempted so that yet a lower level of cream again is needed to maintain skin control. The ultimate aim is to use only a moisturizer to keep the skin soft and supple and prevent unnecessary irritation.

While continuing to pay attention to skin care, it is worth looking at the dietary aspect, and here the approach is in three stages. (Do remember that mild eczema can often be kept under complete control with the use of a low-strength hydrocortisone cream. This is safe and effective, and does away with the need to play around with diets.)

The sequence for troublesome eczema is as follows:

Stage 1 diet: Eliminate cow's milk, eggs and artificial colours/preservatives

Stage 2 diet: Eliminate cow's milk, beef, eggs, chicken and artificial colours/preservatives

Stage 3 diet: Eliminate cow's milk, beef, eggs, chicken, artificial colours/preservatives, nuts, tomatoes and fish

This approach calls for the elimination of most of the offending foods, some of which act as initial sensitizers while others act as aggravators of the condition.

The allergens entering by the respiratory tract can be blocked by the use of aerosol sprays such as are used in asthma and rhinitis (see Chapter 2). The most successful results appear to be gained from the use of Beconase intranasally.

The management of atopic eczema

Because of the complex nature of atopic eczema and the potential problem of under-treating, it is important not to underestimate the need for control. Perhaps the most logical and successful approach is a combination of diet and regular skin care. The difficulty lies in the restrictive diets: how to make the child's meals varied and nutritious yet at the same time not deficient in the substances necessary for growth and development.

My own policy in dealing with troublesome eczema is to recommend the following dietary changes. Remove cow's milk, eggs, chocolate, colourings/preservatives, nuts and tomatoes from the diet. Also, use an anti-allergy preparation called Nalcrom (sodium cromoglycate: in different preparations this is used also in the treatment of asthma and allergic rhinitis) to block any potential allergic mechanisms occurring with other foods. Nalcrom is safe and can be used for months on end; however, it may not work for every child.

In addition to this diet I suggest an adequate and consistent policy on skin care using the 'step-ladder' reducing-strength format. For children left with dry, sensitive skin after this approach it is worth considering the oral use of evening primrose oil (Efamol). This contains essential fatty acids in which eczema patients may be deficient. The addition of evening primrose oil to the diet appears to 'oil the skin from within', and it can make the texture more soft and supple and less sensitive.

There are other factors which irritate eczematous skin and are important in day-to-day control:

Cotton always next to skin
Wool never next to skin
Keep adequate temperatures – never overheat
Maintain bedroom dust-free (see Chapter 7)

Avoid domestic pets
Keep moulds and fungi under control in the house
Avoid soaps/detergents
Keep fingernails trimmed
If possible, use soft water to wash your child

Atopic eczema can be managed through a combination of the dietary approach and the careful control of skin symptoms through the use of adequate strengths of cortisone creams. Nalcrom and evening primrose oil may well be useful in treating selected children, depending on their age and skin condition. Antihistamines are useful for children suffering from a persistent itch.

5

Allergies of the Gastro-Intestinal Tract

For practical purposes, the gastro-intestinal tract begins in the mouth and ends at the rectum. It includes the gullet, stomach and loops of bowel which interconnect and have different functions in the digestive process. Allergy problems can affect this system at any point and produce a variety of symptoms.

A classic example of this is the series of reactions brought about by an egg allergy. Within minutes to an hour of egg ingestion there can be vomiting – often of a vigorous nature. This is followed first by abdominal pains and then by diarrhoea. Here, the sensitivity has produced responses in the stomach (vomiting), upper bowel (abdominal pains) and lower bowel (diarrhoea). Other foods capable of producing similar quick-onset symptoms include peanuts, fish and cow's milk.

The following list includes the majority of symptoms in children that can be caused by allergies – almost exclusively food allergies:

Mouth	Lips tingling and swelling
	Inside of mouth tingling and swelling
	Tongue swelling
	Mouth ulcers
Stomach	Heartburn
(gastritis)	Dyspepsia
	Vomiting
Bowel	Abdominal pains
(colitis)	Diarrhoea
	Blood-stained diarrhoea
	Flatulence
Bowel	Colic
(enteropathy)	Abdominal distension
	Loose stools
	Constipation

Rectum	Anal soreness and eczema
(proctitis)	

These may be accompanied by anaemia, poor weight gain and generalized lethargy.

Some of these symptoms appear so soon after the offending food has been consumed that the diagnosis is clear. Other symptoms are delayed for many hours, which makes for a complicated detection routine.

In children, the commonest foods to produce allergic reactions affecting the gastro-intestinal tract include: cow's milk, egg (usually the white only), cheese, wheat, chocolate, fish (especially shellfish), nuts (especially peanuts), tomatoes, strawberries, citrus fruits, yeasts and spices.

The earliest symptoms occur in infancy, generally in response to cow's milk. There is vomiting, colic, irritability and constipation or diarrhoea. Even exclusively breast-fed babies do not escape, as the offending milk protein can be passed from mother to child via the breast milk.

Other problems make themselves known (or existing problems are made worse) when the child is weaned or when mixed feeding is introduced. If the child has a milk intolerance and continues to take milk, the symptoms can worsen, going, say, from loose stools to diarrhoea or even to blood-stained diarrhoea. Further feeding can cause anaemia, poor weight gain and general irritability.

In an older child, the symptoms of mouth ulcers, dyspepsia, abdominal pains and distension may reflect a continuing food allergy affecting the gastro-intestinal tract.

Elizabeth was breast-fed from birth until the age of six months. In her early months her mother noted bouts of irritability, colic and regurgitation of feeds. These seemed to come in bursts every week – and usually occurred on Mondays. After six months she was weaned on to a milk formula – and the difficulties began almost immediately. First of all she vomited most of her feeds, and then had screaming fits where she could not be pacified. She became constipated.

The doctor diagnosed colic and prescribed an antispasmodic mixture as well as a mild laxative. After a week on these Elizabeth showed no improvement; indeed, she was obviously becoming worse as she had lost weight and looked miserable. A weekend of screaming, irritability and vomiting, and an urgent request from the family doctor, led to her being seen by a paediatrician.

He suspected a milk allergy and put Elizabeth on a special formula which is used in this condition. Within forty-eight hours she was looking happier and less irritable: her feeds stayed down. The colic settled after three days, and on the fourth she passed a normal stool. Elizabeth stayed on her specially modified formula, gaining weight and becoming more like a healthy, happy baby.

The most interesting part of her story was the weekly episode of colic, irritability and regurgitation which had occurred while she was being breast-fed. It transpired that her mother had a strong dislike of cow's milk and had declared herself 'allergic to it' many years previously. However, because she was breast-feeding and concerned about her own nutrition she forced herself to drink two pints of milk every Saturday and Sunday. In all probability this found its way into the breast milk – and into Elizabeth, who produced her symptoms on Mondays!

Allergic symptoms in children tend to become less frequent as they grow older. Most allergies have died down within three years of being diagnosed, with the exception of those related to egg-white, fish and nuts.

Management

Ideally, this means identifying and removing the foods to which the child is allergic. In the case of small babies, this is a relatively easy task as they derive most of their nourishment from milk.

As many as seven per cent of all children are allergic to cow's milk. Such children tend to have a family history of asthma, eczema, hay fever and other allergies: it is claimed that sixty per cent of them have a history of allergies on either one or both sides of the family. When it comes to diagnosis, the sequence of events leading up to the onset of the symptoms is more helpful than the use of investigative procedures. Symptoms which appear after feeding and are similar to those described in the case of Elizabeth are very suggestive of a cow's milk allergy.

The simplest and most reliable method of treating – and, indirectly, of diagnosing – is to remove all milk products and substitute either a soya milk or modified milk formula. (The most popular soya formulas are Wysoy, Formula S and Prosobee; modified milk formulas include Pregistimil and Nutramigen.) This usually leads to the symptoms being resolved, and allows the child to regain health. A small number of children may have problems with even the soya formulas and settle only on one of the modified preparations, which unfortunately, are expensive.

A distinction should be made here between cow's milk allergy and a condition known as lactose intolerance. Lactose is a sugar found in milk. It breaks down in the small intestine into galactose and glucose, which are then absorbed. The breakdown requires the help of an enzyme known as lactase. If this is absent, lactose passes freely into the large intestine, resulting in loose stools, excess wind and a bad nappy rash. The symptoms are similar to those of cow's milk allergy.

Lactase deficiency may be inherited, and occurs particularly often among certain ethnic groups. Inherited lactase deficiency is a lifelong problem. A lesser form of lactase deficiency can occur on a temporary basis in a child who is recovering from gastro-enteritis. Here the story is usually a straightforward one: the child was able to tolerate milk products before the episode of gastro-enteritis but later developed symptoms on taking milk. A fortnight on a diet that excludes all milk products should put an end to this temporary milk intolerance.

In the case of older children on a varied diet where the story and symptoms suggest a food allergy, two kinds of approach are useful:

Stage 1: Eliminate the foods which have been shown by previous experience to cause problems, in other words the most notorious symptom-producing foods. This should include milk and eggs at least.

Stage 2: Subject the child to an 'elimination and challenge' procedure (see Chapter 7).

The latter is a potentially hazardous process and one that should only be authorized and supervised by an experienced doctor. Some children have been known to have dramatic reactions when, after a temporary withdrawal, they are 'challenged' with foods to which they are allergic. Such reactions tend to occur within twenty minutes – sometimes even in seconds – and can lead to collapse, respiratory distress, vomiting, muscular cramps and diarrhoea, sometimes with blood. This practice is not one to be undertaken lightly.

In the case of breast-feeding mothers who suspect their child's symptoms are due to cow's milk intolerance, a milk-free diet should be adhered to for at least five days before total clearance can be expected.

If there is the possibility of multiple food sensitivity, then the anti-allergy preparation Nalcrom can be used. This blocks allergic reactions to certain foods and may permit more varied diet.

Many children with clearly proven food sensitivities grow out of their intolerance in time. It is better to allow at least one year free of the symptom-producing foods if the overall condition is a severe one, for instance in the case of atopic eczema.

Gluten intolerance – coeliac disease

In addition to the problems described, a condition known as coeliac disease is caused by a sensitivity in the bowel to certain foodstuffs. In this case the culprit is gluten, a component of many cereals. Gluten is found in wheat, rye, etc., but not in rice. When eaten it causes damage to the lower bowel lining so that other foods cannot be adequately digested. Children with this sensitivity do not develop symptoms until cereals are introduced to the diet, usually after two months of age. In its most obvious format, gluten sensitivity causes foul smelling diarrhoea, swollen tummy, poor appetite and poor growth. The child may be anaemic (i.e., have a low blood count).

Unfortunately coeliac disease does not always begin with these classic features and many children go undiagnosed for years. These children may have vague symptoms of loose stools, occasional tummy pains and generalized lethargy. More often than not the correct diagnosis is made by chance.

The most important test to confirm coeliac disease involves examining the lining of the bowel under a microscope. While the child is taking gluten products the bowel will look abnormal and only return to a healthy pattern when gluten is removed from the diet. Occasionally milk products are also forbidden as the damaged bowel lining cannot handle one of the sugars present in milk. As soon as the bowel is back to normal, milk can be reintroduced and tolerated.

Gluten sensitivity is a lifelong problem and one that children do not 'grow out of'. Fortunately there are many commercial gluten-free products available so that the diet is not tedious and unexciting.

In addition to coeliac disease, it is possible that a gluten sensitivity may be responsible for a range of other vague symptoms in children, such as mouth ulcers. However, there is no firm proof of this suspicion at present.

6

Miscellaneous Allergies of Children

Arthritis

This is painful, swollen joints especially of the lower limbs. It is possible that a small but significant percentage of children with persistent arthritis may respond to a diet free of dairy produce (from milk). Do remember that there are other causes of arthritis in children — especially infections. No child should be treated by dietary methods alone unless a paediatrician has first made a thorough investigation.

Arthralgia

This consists of aching joints without any obvious sign of inflammation. There are also children who have recurring pains in their limbs – often incorrectly referred to as 'growing pains' – which disappear when an anti-allergy diet is introduced. In fact, there is no such condition as growing pains.

Unexplained fevers (pyrexia)

There are some children who run high temperatures and look unwell on a recurring basis without an exact diagnosis ever being reached. In a recent trial of diet and epilepsy, a number of children developed fevers after being 'challenged' with certain foods as part of the investigation. It appears that food allergy may well be the cause of recurring fevers in some such cases. Again, it is essential that other causes are eliminated before food intolerance is considered.

Bladder problems (eneuresis)

In particular these consist of frequency of passing urine, discomfort on passing urine and difficulty in staying dry (i.e. wetting the bed, wetting the pants) at an age when it is reasonable to expect toilet-training to have been completed. Some children in this situation respond to dietary manipulation, but as a rule they also have other allergy-related problems, such as migraine, over-activity and eczema. The bladder problems are rarely the sole features of an allergic disorder.

Eye symptoms

Pupil abnormalities and blurred vision are the most frequent eye symptoms associated with allergic problems – mainly due to foods. Parents often comment that their children look 'glassy-eyed' if they break their diets by taking foodstuffs to which they react. This is particularly noticeable in the case of hyperactive children.

Nephritis

In simple terms this can be considered an inflammation of the kidneys, and it is a very serious illness. The main features here include swelling of the skin around the eyes, puffiness of the ankles and weight gain due to fluid retention. Protein is found in the urine – it is not usually present there – and special testing reveals abnormal changes in the kidney tissue.

There are certain significant causes of nephritis in children, none of which involve allergic mechanisms. However, reports have been made of allergic reactions to milk and pork definitely leading to nephritis. Such reactions are quite rare compared to the usual, easily identified causes of the condition.

Anaphylactic shock

This is an extreme allergic reaction which develops rapidly and explosively after the exposure to an allergic substance. The features include: generalized itching, faintness, heavy perspiration, nausea/vomiting, extreme shortness of breath, a drop in blood pressure and collapse. *This is a potentially life-threatening condition and one which requires urgent medical attention.*

The causes include bee stings, certain drugs (such as penicillin) and certain foods. One of the commonest foods to provoke such a reaction is shellfish, but others include soya milk and cow's milk. Most of the reactions occur within minutes of ingestion, but occasionally hours may elapse before any symptoms appear.

This is one of the main reasons why parents should be extremely careful when trying out 'elimination and challenge' diets on their children (see Chapter 7). Indeed, such procedures should really only be attempted after consultation with a doctor.

Except in the cases of nephritis and anaphylaxis, the symptoms described in this chapter generally form part of an overall picture of allergy: in other words, the children concerned do not have them in isolation but together with other allergic features such as asthma, rhinitis, eczema and so on. The management of these calls for the same approach as that outlined in other sections of this book, and involves the identification and removal of the offending foodstuffs.

7

The Management of
Allergic Disorders

Inhaled (airborne) allergens

These are the most frequent offenders as far as the allergic disorders of children are concerned, and include: house dust, house-dust mites, feathers, animal danders, hay, straw, moulds and pollens. It is important to identify which substances are involved so that appropriate measures can be taken to deal with the disorder.

The simplest, safest and most effective way of pinpointing these individual allergens is by skin-prick testing. This involves placing drops of extract containing the allergen being tested on the patient's forearm and pricking the skin underneath. In this way a small amount of the extract is allowed to seep beneath the skin surface. A positive result will be shown if the skin starts to itch and a 'weal and flare' reaction occurs: this means that the skin around the extract swells up like a blister and reddens.

Once the allergen has been identified, management of the disorder calls for one of the following methods of approach, which can sometimes be combined:

1 *Identification and avoidance.* An example of this is horsehair allergy. Stay away from horses, stables and any furniture with horsehair stuffing.
2 *Identification and reduction of the allergy load.* This applies, for instance, to the allergy caused by the house-dust mite. As this allergen is impossible to avoid in practical terms, the main thrust of management is directed at reducing the quantity of house-dust mites in the home environment, especially in the bedroom.
3 *Identification and desensitization.* A case in point is the allergy caused by grass pollen. As it is impossible to avoid pollen in the summer months, decisions must be made on

treatment. Many children get fed up with using medication and opt for a desensitization procedure instead (see below).

4   *Pre-treatment.* This implies that the allergens are known and appropriate medication can be taken before exposure. An example of this is Rynacrom (sodium cromoglycate), which can be used for allergic summer rhinitis before the child goes out in the morning at the height of summer.

5   *Treatment on an SOS basis.* In other words, use medicine only when the symptoms appear. An example of this would be a Stage 1 bronchodilator for the child who wheezes only on exposure to dust, and infrequently at that.

6   *Treatment on a regular basis.* An example of this would be persistent asthma requiring long-term medication.

Taking allergic asthma as an example, it may be useful to combine approaches 1, 2, 3 and 5 as follows:

Identify and avoid allergens wherever possible.
Identify and reduce other allergen loads.
Identify and desensitize in the case of a very troublesome single allergen.
Treat on an SOS basis for occasional allergen exposure.

Now let us look at the most common inhaled/airborne allergens and see what in practical terms can be done to reduce exposure to them.

House dust/house-dust mite

This is a tiny insect – so minute that it can be seen only with the aid of a microscope – which lives in and feeds off the many substances found in household dust. Dust mites live in dust, so this must be removed from those rooms which the child frequents – especially the bedroom. In particular, the mite thrives in carpets, curtains and the seams of mattresses.

Here are some suggestions for dealing with the problem:

Use only synthetic bedding materials.
Wash all sheets every week.
Avoid feathers, down, or flock in bedding materials.

Get blankets/duvets/mattresses into the sun as often as possible.

Vacuum more often than usual, paying attention to under the bed, the curtains and even the mattress.

Put clothes away in wardrobes and keep soft toys in a playroom. Do not leave dressing gowns behind doors.

Use lightweight curtain materials and wash them every six weeks.

In the case of severe allergic conditions consider changing carpets for vinyl.

Treat the mattress with a spray called Tymasil to kill off the house-dust mite population.

Cover the mattress with a plastic sheet.

These measures will dramatically reduce the amount of exposure received to dust and dust mites.

Feathers

If your child is allergic to feathers, remove feather-filled pillows and duvets, replacing these with synthetic filled duvets and pillows.

Animal danders

No pet should be allowed into the bedroom of an allergic child. If there are furry pets – and this category ranges from dogs to hamsters – decisions may have to be made as to where they are allowed in the house, who cleans the cage, and so on. If the pets are allowed to sleep in the living-room, it is important that their dander is vacuumed away quickly. If you have an allergic child and are contemplating buying a pet, the best advice is 'Don't'. Try and persuade him or her to make friends with goldfish – at least they don't shed hair!

Pollens

Large quantities of pollen are produced by trees, grasses, rushes and weeds. The first tree to pollinate is the hazel – in February – followed by a regular succession of others until June. Most weed pollen is released mainly between June and July. A lawn grass, *Poa annua*, produces pollen from March to September, and its pollen is released every time the grass is cut.

Pollens need dry conditions for release: dew or rain damps down pollination. Rain, especially drizzle, washes the air clean of pollen. Warm air speeds up pollination, so calm, sunny days produce high yields of pollen. In the country, pollen is released in mid morning and peaks at 'nose level' in the afternoon. In cities, the pollen peak is delayed until after sunset. The sea coast is a refuge for pollen allergy victims, unless there is a land-to-sea wind; during the day most wind directions are sea-to-land, but at night this is reversed.

Not a great deal can be done to avoid pollens, but a few simple tips are worth mentioning:

Shut windows on car/train journeys.

Avoid parks and fields on high-pollen-count days.

Moulds

Mould spores come into the air in large numbers in late summer. The same rules apply to mould allergy as to pollen allergy. Mould sufferers should keep well away from harvesting areas.

Hay/straw

Avoidance is the only practical advice that can be given, apart from pre-treatment, which is a sensible precaution for those who cannot get away from such areas.

Desensitization

This is a routine where, over a number of weeks, a series of injections are given which help stimulate the body into coping better with inhaled allergens. It works well when individual allergens can be identified and fit in with the condition, for instance in the case of the grass pollens that produce summer 'hay fever'. The main failures here relate to attempts to use too many allergens in the desensitization vaccine. To achieve the best results the technique should be monitored by testing the nose and chest at the end of the schedule for signs of responsiveness to the substances being tested. A reduced or poor response – for instance, no wheezing or sneezing – suggests the technique is working. The routine works well for pollen and house-dust mite allergies.

Food allergens

While there are many different foods which can cause allergic problems in children, a certain number of these keep turning up as the culprits in the majority of conditions. These include cow's milk, eggs, citrus fruits, chocolate, artificial colourings and preservatives, fish, nuts (especially peanuts) and tomatoes.

The suspicion that milk may be involved in any allergic condition is raised if the following features were present when in infancy the child was fed a milk formula:

Persistent vomiting
Colic
Constipation/diarrhoea
Nasal or chest excess mucus
Irritability
Eczema
Wheezing

In the case of other foods being involved, suspicion is raised by the condition itself and by its response to dietary elimination. Two approaches can be followed which are based on diet alone:

1 Eliminate those foods which have been shown by previous experience to be most troublesome in individual conditions.
2 Perform an 'elimination and challenge' routine. Here, the child is put on those foods least likely to cause allergies and one by one other foods are introduced into the diet. Any reactions are recorded so that at the end of the test, in theory, it should be possible to have identified which are responsible for the allergic condition.

The practical difficulties connected with this exercise are many, and include the following:

It involves putting the child on a very restricted diet which is bound to be deficient in basic nutrients.

The possible misinterpretation of reactions.

The possible confusion involved when it comes to deciding which foods cause which response (some produce immediate reactions, whereas other reactions may not show anything for up to seventy-two hours).

The risk of a severe reaction to certain foods in the case of highly allergic children.

The foods *least* likely to cause allergies are as follows:

Meat: lamb
Cereal: rice
Vegetable: peeled potatoes
            carrots
            lettuce
Fruit: pears
Fat: a refined vegetable seed oil, such as sunflower oil
Drink: spring water and sugar

It should be noted that on an elimination diet symptoms often get worse before they begin to get better. In this context, an initial exacerbation of the condition may actually be a good sign.

New foods should be added every three to seven days and taken in reasonable quantities. If this procedure is followed through accurately, the child will end up with a list of foods which do not cause allergic reactions and, hopefully, allow for an adequate, varied and nutritious diet.

Some doctors recommend 'rotating' the safe foods so that the child does not end up becoming allergic to even these. This means that the diet is varied on a day-to-day basis and that the same foods are not taken repetitively. For highly allergic children in whom many foods produce reactions, this 'rotation' of diet is probably a good idea.

My own policy is to avoid 'elimination and challenge' routines and to use instead diets which cut out the known most troublesome foods in individual conditions. In addition, I recommend the use of Nalcrom (sodium cromoglycate) to block the possible allergic reactions of other foods in the diet. Nalcrom is an anti-allergy preparation which works for some children with food allergies. It is swallowed before meals.

Alternative methods of diagnosis and treatment

Useful tests

Blood tests. As a general rule, blood tests are not terribly helpful in the management of allergies in children. The tests may show a very allergic nature (a raised IgE), but this is usually obvious from simple observation. (IgE, immunoglobulin E, is one of the antibodies thought to play a major role in allergies.) A different test, called the RAST, is used as a means of identifying the specific allergens involved in individual conditions. This test is quite expensive, and no more accurate than skin-testing. RAST test results take two or three days to become available, whereas skin tests can be read within thirty to forty minutes.

Tests of doubtful value

Pulse testing. This relies on the measurement of a rise in pulse after the patient has consumed something likely to cause an allergic reaction. It is open to so many variables that it is of no practical use.

Basophil degranulation test. This still requires evaluation.

Sublingual drop test. Diluted solutions of the foods to be tested are placed under the tongue and the patient observed for any allergic reactions. This is an extremely imperfect test and one that is of no use in practical terms.

Cytotoxic testing. A diagnosis of allergy is suggested if a food solution is added to a blood sample and the white cells are observed to die. This test is time-consuming, gives false positives and is considered inaccurate so often as to be useless in diagnosis.

Intradermal testing. A deeper form of skin-prick testing, this carries a small risk of producing a severe allergic reaction. Too many false positives occur with this test for it to be considered useful in diagnosis.

Useless tests

Hair analysis. This test involves having a hair sample analysed by a private laboratory. This will not detect any form of allergy, and it also produces widely differing results (even from the same head!) when used in testing for trace-metal deficiencies.

Radionics, radiesthesia, psionic medicine and dowsing. Such practices are ineffective when it comes to diagnosing or treating allergies in children.

Dangerous advice and practices

Occasionally children are subjected by their parents to various diets and other forms of treatment which are likely to cause harm. Almost exclusively, the children concerned have allergy-related problems. These are the most frequently encountered nowadays.

Autoimmune urine therapy. Here, the patient is made to drink his or her own urine. Apart from the obvious unpleasantness involved, this practice is a potentially dangerous one.

Macrobiotic diets. These are likely to give rise to nutritional deficiencies in growing children.

The supplementation of the diet with trace elements. Allergies cannot be cured by vitamin/trace element supplementation. The overuse of vitamin and trace-mineral preparations can actually cause problems in children.

Treatment for intestinal candidiasis. The theory here is that the intestinal tract has been 'taken over' by the growth of an organism called *Candida albicans* (also known as yeast or thrush). Treatment involves low-sugar, low-yeast diets and the use of a powder to kill off the *Candida* in the bowel. Such suggestions and treatments are of no use and only deflect attention away from correct procedures.

8

Allergy Avoidance Diets

The best way to treat an allergic disorder is through identification and, ideally, removal of the offending allergen. In the case of airborne allergens, total avoidance is obviously far from easy (see Chapter 7 for advice on this).

Food allergies are more difficult in that here identification and removal is a less straightforward matter. Foods that produce immediate responses are easy to identify and to avoid, but problems arise when children develop reactions either to several foods or to a common basic food such as milk, which is an ingredient in a wide range of commercially prepared foods.

Not infrequently the reaction is not to all the components of a particular food but to certain parts of it. For example, children tend to be more allergic to egg white than to egg yolk.

Heating or cooking foods may reduce their 'allergicness', but not in every case. Fish, tomatoes and eggs remain just as troublesome from an allergy point of view even after being heated, and the most significant allergic protein in milk is heat-stable. On the other hand some foods have their 'allergicness' reduced through heating or processing: for instance evaporated or long-life milk may be tolerated in certain cases where ordinary pasteurized milk causes reactions.

Furthermore, children vary in the degree to which they are allergic. Some can tolerate butter but not milk, some small amounts of egg in cakes but not in any other form, while others react to even minute traces of the offending foods.

Diets

A Milk-free (could be useful in rhinitis, sinusitis, catarrh, asthma, serous otitis, migraine, epilepsy, hyperactivity, eczema, urticaria, bowel/bladder disorders, arthritis, nephritis)

61

B   Milk-/egg-free (could be useful in eczema, urticaria)

C   Milk-/egg-/colouring- and preservative-free (could be useful in eczema, urticaria)

D   Milk-/egg-/chicken-/beef-/colouring- and preservative-free (could be useful in eczema)

E   Milk-/egg-/chicken-/nut-/tomato-/fish-/colouring- and preservative-free (could be useful in eczema)

F   Milk-/egg-/chocolate-/nut-/tomato-/colouring- and preservative-free, with Nalcrom added (of use *only* in eczema)

G   Azo-dye- and benzoate-free (could be useful in nasal polyps, hyperactivity, urticaria)

H   Salicylate-free (useful in hyperactivity, nasal polyps)

I   Colouring- and preservative-free (useful in hyperactivity, asthma, eczema, urticaria)

J   Sulphite-free (useful in asthma)

K   Yeast-free (useful in asthma)

A   *Milk-free*

The following are forbidden: milk; cream; cheese; butter; ordinary margarine; galactomins and products containing casein; whey milk solids; milk puddings (such as custard); creamed rice; baby cereals fortified with milk solids; Horlicks, Ovaltine, etc.; all types of ice cream; chocolate (unless milk-free); cream tinned and packet soups. Granose or white Flora margarine can be used in this diet. Granose is a vegetable margarine containing animal products. It is gluten free, lactose free, additive free and available in health food shops or some supermarkets.

B   *Milk-/egg-free*

As above, with the following also being forbidden: eggs (including omelettes, meringues, etc.); tinned and processed foods containing egg.

C   *Milk-/egg-/artificial colouring- and preservative-free*

As A and B, with the following also being forbidden: azo-dyes;

salicylates (see diets G and H); tartrazine E102*; sunset yellow E110*; new coccine (E124)*; oil of wintergreen; yellow food dyes; benzoate and benzoic acid (E210–219) inclusive; all syrups and some vitamin medicines; coloured sweets and tablets (especially orange, red, green or yellow ones); coloured toothpastes.

Food labels which state 'permitted preservative or colouring' should *not* be given. Check every food package before giving any item. Watch out especially for: supermarket-packaged meats; fish fingers; canned meats and fish; flavoured milks; coloured cheeses; packaged soups; flavoured foods; flavoured crisps and chips; fruit squashes and fizzy drinks; cordials; lozenges and cough syrups; most confectionery, sauces; pickles; jams, etc. unless homemade.

Use only white toothpaste.

D   Milk-/egg-/chicken-/beef-/colouring- and preservative-free

As A, B and C, with the further elimination of chicken and beef, also of chicken/beef stocks and flavourings, etc.

E   Milk-/egg-/chicken-/nut-/tomato-/fish-/colouring- and preservative-free

As C, with the additional elimination of chicken, nuts, tomatoes and fish. This includes tomato ketchup and flavourings, fish pastes, chicken stocks and all forms of nuts and nut oils.

F   Milk-/egg-/chocolate-/nut-/tomato-/colouring- and preservative-free, with Nalcrom added

As C, with the further elimination of chocolate, nuts and tomatoes. In addition the anti-allergy preparation Nalcrom (sodium cromoglycate) is taken to block the potential reactions of other foods.

---

* E102 etc. correspond to the serial numbers used on food labels as alternatives to the specific names of additives. (See also Appendix 5.)

G   Azo-dye- and benzoic acid-free

The following are forbidden: white flour (except unbleached from health food shops); soft drinks; salami, sausage, paté; smoked fish; some tinned foods; preservatives and confectionery, especially tartrazine (orange yellow) E102, sunset yellow E110, new coccine E124 and the preservatives E210–E219; vegetables and fruits rich in salicylates, such as rhubarb, bananas and peas; aspirin and medicines containing aspirin which may be labelled sodium salicylate (this is due to a cross-sensitivity between salicylates and the azo-dyes/benzoic acid preservatives); medicinal syrups and coloured tablets, especially orange, red, green and yellow (sugar-coated tablets and capsules may be taken); antihistamine syrups and tablets (but the following are allowed: Dimotane, Fabahistin, Tavegil, Phenergan, Atarax, Optimine). Other medicines, toothpastes, vitamin preparations, pastilles and lozenges containing synthetic flavouring and colourings should be avoided.

H   Salicylate-free

Salicylates are found in aspirin and aspirin-containing medicines, which may be labelled 'acetylsalicylic acid'. The following also have a high content of natural salicylate: dried fruits; berry fruits; oranges; apricots; pineapples; cucumbers; gherkins; endive; olives; grapes; almonds; liquorice; peppermint; honey; many herbs and spices, including thyme, mint, paprika, rosemary, oregano and curry; tomato sauce, Worcester sauce; tea; wines, including port; liqueurs.

Children with a definite salicylate sensitivity should avoid the following commonly prescribed medications as they may produce cross-sensitivity reactions: Indocid (indomethacin); Naprosyn (naproxen); Brufen (ibuprofen); Ponstan (mefenamic acid); Clinoril (sulindac); Fenopron/Progesic (fenoprofen).

If analgesics (painkillers) are required, then plain paracetamol (such as Panadol) should be used.

I   Colouring- and preservative-free

As G, also eliminating foods likely to contain tartrazine, which include: fruit squashes and cordials; coloured fizzy drinks;

pickles; bottled sauces; salad cream; shop-bought cakes; cake mix; soups (packets and tins); custard; instant puddings; coloured sweets; filled chocolates; jelly; ice cream and lollies; jam; marmalade; curry powder; mustard; yoghurt.

Tartrazine is water-soluble and gives a pleasant lemon yellow colour to foods. It is also used in some medicine capsules. The incidence of sensitivity is between one in ten thousand and one in a thousand.

J   Sulphite-free

The food preservatives sulphur dioxide and sodium metabisulphite can aggravate asthma in susceptible children. Such children are sensitive to the irritant effect of sulphur dioxide gas which is liberated from sodium metabisulphite in acid foods and inhaled in low concentrations during eating. The following are the foods and drinks often involved in sulphite reactions: food prepared for use in the catering trade (such as prepared salads, avocado dip, potatoes, shrimps); dehydrated fruits (such as dried apricots, apples, peaches, pears and other blanched fruits); fruit products (concentrates, syrups, purées, jams); dehydrated vegetables (such as dried carrots, potatoes, cabbage, dehydrated meals for campers and hikers, soup mixes); raw vegetables (cut potatoes for French fries); shrimps; wine (especially homemade and foreign wines); beer; fruit juices; orange drinks; powdered milk.

K   Yeast-free

Yeast allergy is more common in adults than in children, and usually produces wheezing. Yeast is found in Marmite, Oxo, Bovril and Bisto. Many foods contain yeast as a flavouring agent, frequently described as a 'flavouring agent' or as 'hydrolysed protein'.

Glossary of medical terms

Adenoids   A small mass of soft tissue located at the back of the throat.

Allergy   Tissue sensitivity to certain substances.

Allergen   Any substance capable of producing an allergic reaction.

Allergic reaction   An abnormal response to a substance tolerated well by normal (i.e. non-allergic) individuals.

Angio-oedema   An allergic condition in which there is either transient or persistent swelling of areas on the skin. The swelling is accompanied by an intense itch and may distort the sufferer's normal features considerably.

Antibodies   (in relation to allergy): One of the defence proteins released to deal with allergens gaining entry to the body.

Antihistamines   One of the hormones released in allergy is called histamine. It is responsible for many of the symptoms (such as the itch). Drugs which block the effects of histamine are called antihistamines.

Arthritis   An inflammation of the bony joints in the body.

Artificial colourings/preservatives   Substances used in food processing to prolong shelf life and make foodstuffs look appetising.

Asthma   A label used to describe the collection of symptoms of coughing, wheezing and shortness of breath.

Atopic   (as in an 'atopic person') An inherited tendency to develop allergy.

Bronchodilator   Drug used to relieve bronchospasm (see the next term).

Bronchospasm   A narrowing of the air tubes (bronchi) of the lungs. This is the major feature in asthma.

Bronchi   Medical term used to describe the tubes in the lungs through which air is inhaled and exhaled.

Catarrh   A persistent trickle of mucus down the back of the throat.

Colic   Stomach cramps.

Colitis   Inflammation of the bowel.

Conjunctivitis (*allergic*)   Inflammation of the whites of the eyes.

Danders (*animal*)   A mixture of fur/hair, scale and urine shed from animals.

Dermographism   The phenomenon of being able to 'write' letters on the skin by the use of pressure alone. Itchy weals rise up to form whatever shape is contrived by pressing.

Desensitization   A method of building up resistance to allergens.

Eczema   Descriptive term given to a skin condition in which there is redness, itching, blistering and weeping.

Epilepsy   *Grand mal*: A convulsion associated with unconsciousness, generalized muscle spasm and, often, incontinence; *petit mal*: a temporary loss of concentration which occurs in children. The child may 'turn off' for seconds or minutes and become oblivious to external events.

Enuresis   Wetting at an age beyond which bladder control might be expected to have been achieved.

Enteropathy   Disease of part of the intestinal tract.

Gastritis   Inflammation of the stomach lining.

Grommets   Small tubes inserted into the eardrums to allow adequate ventilation of the inner ear.

Hay fever   Term used to describe a collection of the following symptoms: a blocked, runny and itchy nose; red, itchy, watery eyes; and sneezing.

Histamine   One of the major substances released in allergic reactions and responsible for many of the associated symptoms.

House dust   A mixture of everything likely to produce household dust. Wool is a major component.

House-dust mite   A minute insect that lives in and feeds off the human skin scales present in dust. Allergy occurs to the mite, both alive and dead, and to its excrement.

Hyperactivity   A poorly defined and much abused label used to describe an abnormal behaviour pattern in children.

Inflammation (*allergic*)   The response of sensitized tissue to allergens. The tissue swells, secretes mucus and often itches.

IgE   The antibody most involved in allergy.

Moulds   Fungi which grow in damp conditions.

Migraine   A specific type of headache.

Nebulizer   An electrically powered unit which pumps liquid medication into a fine mist which can then be breathed in.

Nephritis   An inflammation of the kidney.

Ocular   Related to the eye.

Polyp   The end-product of persistent swelling of the sinus tissue with protrusion into the nose. It is a grape-like structure causing blockage, loss of smell, and restricted air entry.

Proctitis   Inflammation of the rectum.

Pyrexia   Fever.

Pollen   The fertilizing powder formed in flowers.

RAST   A test used in allergy.

Rhinitis   Inflammation of the nose.

Sinusitis   Inflammation of the sinuses.

Steroid   One of the cortisone-based drugs.

Tearing   Excess shedding of tears (watery eyes).

Tension/fatigue syndrome   Medical jargon for being 'run-down'.

Thrush   Also known as *Monilia* or *Candida*. A fungal infection which causes a white, cheesy substance to form on tissue.

Turbinates   Ridges of tissue that line part of the nose.

Wheeze   A musical sound, rather like that of an organ or whistle, coming from the chest and usually occurring in asthma.

Appendix 2

List of Conditions due to Allergy, with Causes and Treatments

Condition	Allergen(s)	Diet(s) (see Chapter 8)
Conjunctivitis	Airborne	Not applicable
Rhinitis	Airborne±foods	A
Sinusitis	Airborne±foods	B
Polyps	Airborne±foods	G, H minimum
Catarrh	Foods?	A?
Asthma	Airborne±foods	All diets possible
Asthma/eczema/polyps	Foods	G, H minimum
Serous otitis	Airborne±foods	A
Migraine	Foods	All diets possible except J, K
Epilepsy	Foods	All diets possible except J, K
Hyperactivity	Usually foods	All diets possible except J, K
Tension/fatigue syndrome	Airborne±foods	All diets possible
Atopic eczema	Airborne±foods± contact	A through to F

Condition	Allergen(s)	Diet(s) (see Chapter 8)
Urticaria/angio-oedema	Foods ± contact	G, H minimum
Hay fever	Airborne	Not applicable
Mouth ulcers	Foods	All diets possible except J, K
Abdominal pains/ discomfort/distension	Foods	All diets possible except J, K
Bowel disturbances (constipation/diarrhoea/ perianal soreness)	Foods	Mainly A
Arthritis	Foods	A if at all
Arthralgia	Foods	All diets possible except J, K
Unexplained fevers (pyrexia)	Foods	All diets possible except J, K
Bladder problems	Foods	All diets possible except J, K
Eye symptoms	Foods	All diets possible except J, K
Nephritis	Foods	Only very rarely milk and pork

Appendix 3

Drugs Used in the Management
of Asthma

In Chapter 2, I explained the sequence of changes which occurs in asthma. It is worth recalling the following:

Normal air tube ⟶   Stage 1: Narrowed air tube (bron-
(bronchus)   choconstriction)
                         ↓
                         Stage 2: Further narrowing due to
                         the combination of muscle
                         contraction and swelling of inner
                         lining of the lung tubes
                         ↓
                         Stage 3: As Stages 1 and 2, with the
                         addition of mucus production and
                         secretion into air tube

Listed below are the drugs most commonly prescribed to reverse the Stage 1 sequence. I have given them under their usual trade names, types of preparation and potential side-effects.

Drug name	Preparation	Possible side-effect(s)
Alupent	Tablet, syrup, aerosol, injection, expectorant	Rapid heartbeat, nausea
Atrovent	Aerosol, nebulizer solution	Unpleasant taste
Berotec	Aerosol, nebulizer solution	Palpitations

Drug name	Preparation	Possible side-effect(s)
Bricanyl	Tablet, syrup, inhaler, injection	Irritant effect of inhaler may cause coughing
Duovent	Aerosol	Rapid heartbeat
Exirel	Capsule, syrup, inhaler	Rapid heartbeat
Nuelin*	Tablet, liquid	Nausea, depression
Phyllocontin*	Tablet	Nausea, depression, aching limbs, stomach-ache
Pulmadil	Inhaler	Palpitations
Slo-Phyllin*	Capsule	Nausea, depression, aching limbs, stomach-ache
Theo-Dur*	Tablet	Nausea, depression, aching limbs, stomach-ache
Theograd*	Tablet	Nausea, depression, aching limbs, stomach-ache
Theolan*	Capsule	Nausea, depression, aching limbs, stomach-ache
Uniphyllin*	Tablet	Nausea, depression, aching limbs, stomach-ache

* In toxic doses these drugs can cause convulsions in children. Their level in the blood is usually monitored by regular sampling.

Drug name	Preparation	Possible side-effect(s)
Ventolin	Syrup, tablets, inhaler, rotacaps, nebulizer solution, injection	Palpitations, rapid heartbeat

Drugs used to reverse stages 2 and 3 in the asthma sequence

(a) By inhalation:

Drug name	Preparation	Side-effect
Becotide	Aerosol, rotacap, nebulizer solution	Thrush in the mouth*
Becloforte	Aerosol	Thrush in the mouth*
Bextasol	Aerosol	Thrush in the mouth*
Pulmicort	Aerosol	Thrush in the mouth*

* This side-effect can be minimized by rinsing the mouth with warm water after using the preparation.

(b) By injection: Cordelsol, Decadron, Efcortelan, Kenalog, Depo-Medrone

(c) By tablet: Decadron, Prednisone, Decortisyl, Deltacortril, Prednisolone, Ledercort, Sintisone

Side-effects of long-term cortisone usage

The drugs listed in (b) and (c) above, when used logically and for short periods, do not produce side-effects. However, prolonged use may lead to quite serious problems, including fluid retention, obesity, a 'moon-face', bruising, the slow healing of wounds, the weakening of the bones and interference with natural cortisone production in the body. It is most unusual for children to be on long-term cortisone treatment given by tablet or injection.

Preventive drugs for asthma

Drug	Preparation	Side-effects
Intal	Inhaler, spinhaler, nebulizer solution	Apart from the taste and possible irritant effects producing a cough, this drug is remarkably free of side-effects.

The following drugs are also used as preventives in asthma: Becotide, Becloforte, Bextasol and Pulmicort (see previous section).

Appendix 4

Other Drugs Used in
Allergy Management

Allergic conjunctivitis

In Chapter 1, I described the features of allergic conjunctivitis. The following eye-drops are commonly used to treat this condition:

Drug name	Side-effect
Opticrom	None
Betnesol*/Neo-Cortef*	Cataracts, glaucoma

* There are many kinds of cortisone-based eye-drops, but these are the most commonly prescribed. The side-effects listed will only occur with prolonged usage, which is most unlikely in the case of children.

Allergic rhinitis

In the case of allergic rhinitis, the following nasal sprays are often prescribed:

Drug name	Side-effects
Beconase	Occasional mild bleeding and of nuisance value only

Drug name	Side-effects
Rhinocort	None reported
Syntaris	Very irritating to use and may actually be painful. Makes the eyes water.
Rynacrom/Lomusol	Both are the same but in different preparations. There are no side-effects.

Antihistamines

These are the drugs used to block the effects of the hormone histamine, which is released in many allergic reactions. The list of those available is very long, and the predominant side-effect is drowsiness. There are two fairly new preparations called Triludan and Hismanal, which are quite free of side-effects and appear to be more effective than their older competitors.

Long-acting cortisone preparations

Kenalog and Depo-Medrone are both given by injection and last for up to six weeks. They are used to treat a range of allergies, such as hay fever, asthma and so on on a 'one-off' basis. It is not common practice to use these drugs repeatedly over a long period because of the possible side-effects. (See under 'Long-term cortisone usage' in Appendix 3, p. 73.)

Miscellaneous other drugs

Nalcrom

This is used to block the effects of food allergens, for example in the case of atopic eczema. There are no real side-effects.

OTHER DRUGS USED IN ALLERGY MANAGEMENT

Efamol

This is evening primrose oil, a herbal substance rich in essential fatty acids. This is quite often used in the treatment of eczema and hyperactivity. There are no side-effects.

Tymasil

This is an aerosol spray which kills off house-dust mites. It is used on mattresses, carpets, etc. and does not have side-effects.

Appendix 5
Artificial Colourings and Preservatives

Eighty per cent of the food we eat is processed in one form or another. By this I mean that the food is changed from its original, natural state to that which we buy on the supermarket shelves. In many cases the food has to be processed to be eaten – for example, milling produces flour which in turn is used in the baking of bread; milk is pasteurized and bottled so that a safe product is conveniently available. However, food processing involves a good deal more than these simple examples, so it is useful to have a closer look at the industry.

Foods are processed for the following main reasons:

1   To preserve the food and extend the shelf life. Preservation reduces wastage and cost. It enables us to eat our favourite foods all year round and so enables us to benefit from economies of scale by growing large quantities of food over large areas of suitable land.
2   Processing makes food safe by destroying dangerous organisms and toxins.
3   Processing may improve the attractiveness of food, its flavour or its appearance.
4   Processing provides convenience, and convenient foods relieve much of the drudgery associated with cooking.

Let us look at another example of the need for processing. So-called 'fresh' fruit often comes from half way around the world and has been in storage for weeks. Bananas are picked in the tropics before they are ripe, shipped and stored at a controlled even temperature and ripened by exposure to ethylene gas (which is given off naturally by ripening fruit). Oranges are picked ripe, shipped and stored at a lower temperature in dry air with a raised carbon dioxide level. The skins are protected from mould infections by wrapping with chemically impregnated paper. Although these fruits have been in artificial environments they are intact and alive and their cells are absorbing oxygen and producing carbon dioxide. This is a very acceptable and important form of processing, and one that is unlikely to cause concern.

However, food manufacturers in their desire to supply unusual and innovative food products at a reasonable profit have introduced artificial chemicals into processing. These chemicals have been added in increasing numbers and quantities over the years to a point where serious doubts have been raised about their usefulness and effects on health. These chemicals are known as 'additives' and the type which cause most concern are the colouring and preservative agents. The colouring additives do exactly what their name suggests: they colour foods so that they look more attractive on the shelves and are as close to the natural product colour as possible. For example, many orange drinks only look orange because of a colouring agent. Without it they would be a rather unattractive neutral colour. Packaged bacon would not have the nice 'healthy' colour without the use of artificial colouring. Indeed the colour of packaged bacon without the artificial agent would look so bad as to be considered having 'gone off'.

The number of additives used in food processing is considerable, and new ones are added regularly. All food additives are subject to close scrutiny by the Food Advisory Committee – a group of experts who advise the Minister of Agriculture, Fisheries and Foods, and the Department of Health – and have to meet two essential criteria: are they necessary and are they safe? The safety question is checked by testing the use of the additive in various animal species and then reviewed regularly by food toxicologists. Recent reports have been very critical of these experts and their committees. Unfortunately their dealings are protected by the Official Secrets Act and consequently any investigation of their decisions is necessarily limited. However, the general unease about the safety of food additives has greatly increased and the experts are having to review the situation carefully.

The public demand for healthier, additive-free foods is reflected in the number of products now openly advertised as 'free from artificial colourings and preservatives'. In Britain the Safeway chain of stores has become 'organic' and now stocks only organically grown fruit and vegetables rather than the mass-produced, artificially fertilized and pesticide-sprayed alternatives. This same group removed all unnecessary additives from their produce in 1985 in response to consumer demand. The first products to be modified were those consumed by children.

The additives which are currently in many packaged, tinned, and bottled foods may cause ill health in susceptible people. Whether the reaction to the chemical is due to an allergic response is immaterial – the offending additive has to be avoided. Because of the wide number of chemicals involved it is almost impossible to know for certain which produce harmful effects in children and how or why they occur at all. However, we now know that children with allergies should avoid the following notorious food additives which have been shown to cause problems to others in the past.

E102	Tartrazine (or orange, yellow)	Reactions include asthma, hyperactivity, worsening eczema, and urticaria
E104	Quinoline yellow	
E107	Yellow 2G	
E110	Sunset yellow	
E124	Ponceau 4R	
E127	Erythrosive	
E150	Caramel	
E210–E219	Benzoates or benzoic acid	
E249	Potassium nitrite	Asthma and hyperactivity
E250	Sodium nitrite	
E251	Sodium nitrate	
E320	BHA	Skin rashes, hyperactivity
E321	BHT	
E621/622/623	Monosodium glutamate MSG	Asthma, hyperactivity, skin rashes; often severe reaction involving total body

The 'E' numbers represent the chemicals added in foodstuffs and should be on the labels of whatever packaging or bottling etc. the food is contained. Additives which are mentioned on labels are usually listed according to their function in the food, e.g. preservative, emulsifier, etc. Quite often the exact name of the chemical in question will be replaced by the serial number (or E number) as in 'Preservative E200'.

The rules governing the labelling of foodstuffs are being tightened but at present the situation is most unsatisfactory. Quite often the only thing on the packaging will be 'permitted colouring and flavouring'. This is useless to the mother of an allergic child. The 'permitted' part of the description refers only to the Food Advisory Committee regulations and we know that a number of additives cleared by them are definitely harmful in susceptible children.

The Safeway chain of supermarkets went organic and removed unnecessary additives after pressure from their customers. In particular the Hyperactive Child Support Group advised its members to lobby ceaselessly and complain bitterly about the use of these chemicals in foods. Their success should be a spur to us all to take the issue in hand more forcefully and to demand stricter controls of these chemicals. If you feel strongly enough about this topic then mention it to your supermarket manager as often as you can. Nag your butcher, your baker and anyone else you buy food from to be more aware of the dangers of some of these additives. Something has to be done to bring the food industry to its senses in this regard. You can help by refusing to buy suspect products and buying as fresh and wholesome foods as possible.

If you would like to read more on this subject then I would suggest the following publications:

E for Additives by Maurice Hanssen (Thorsons)
Food Additives – taking the lid off what we really eat by Erik Millstone (Penguin)
Look at the Label A publication by the Ministry of Agriculture, Fisheries and Food which explains what the labels

on pre-packed food mean and why they are important. Copies of this booklet are available free of charge, from HMSO PO Box 569 London SE1 9NH. When ordering remember to ask for any amendments.

Appendix 6

Substitutes for Cow's Milk

Breast milk

This is the perfect infant formula, and in cases where a milk allergy is suspected during breast-feeding it is probably being transmitted by the mother's intake of milk. Only extremely rarely are children allergic to their mother's milk alone.

Goat's milk

This is unsuitable for infants under one year, and is not very different from cow's milk from an allergic point of view: indeed, there have been cases of children becoming allergic to goat's milk after switching from cow's milk. If it is used, the following must be supplemented: vitamins A, C, D, B12 and folic acid.

Soya formulas

There are three excellent soya formulas which can be substituted for cow's milk when allergy to it is confirmed. These are: Wysoy (made by Wyeth Laboratories), Formula S (made by Cow and Gate) and Prosobee (made by Mead and Johnson). All three are lactose-free in order to make them suitable for children with cow's milk intolerance, who are often intolerant to lactose.

Ewe's and other mammalian milks

These tend to be high in energy, protein and fat and low in carbohydrate. They are unsuitable for infants and should only be given to children aged over one year.

Modified milk formulas

There are two formulas which have been modified to make them less allergic and more digestible, and these are: Pregestimil (Mead and Johnson), which is suitable for babies under six months; and Nutramigen (Mead and Johnson), which is better reserved for children over six months of age.

These two preparations are much more expensive than any other milk substitute, but they are available on prescription in the United Kingdom.

Appendix 7

Catering for Food Allergies
Made Easy – by Maura Thornhill

Catering for a child with food allergies is much easier than might first appear. When the allergens are removed from the child's diet, the extent of the improvement can be quite dramatic. The extra effort involved is very worth while.

Parents catering for an allergic child will soon find two powerful factors working in their favour. The first is a far greater public awareness of allergy than was previously the case. This is reflected in the ready availability of a wide variety of 'special' foodstuffs such as soya milk, margarines free of artificial colouring and milk products, additive-free jams and fruit spreads, chocolate substitutes (based on carob), wholemeal fruit bars and special 'sweets' and crisps. This situation contrasts starkly with the position a mere ten years ago: then, a friend of mine recalls, she could only get soya milk on prescription. Today this is stocked by most supermarkets. The increase in the amount of information provided on food labels is also of great assistance.

The second – rather surprising – factor is that the child herself will soon come to associate cause and effect, and with remarkably little encouragement will steer clear of the foods to which she is allergic. This encouraging response can be obtained from even three-year-olds. All that is required are parental encouragement and attractive alternatives to the usual chocolate bars, cakes and so on.

Plan of action

1 Determine which are the foods to which your child is allergic.
2 Compile a short list of permitted foods. This will call for an initial investigation of your local supermarkets, health food and ethnic shops. Read food labels carefully and get to know some of the less familiar terms: for instance, casein and whey

are derivatives of cow's milk; E160 is carotene, a pale yellow colouring. (See Appendix 5 for useful books on additives.)

3 Draw up a menu for the first week. This should help you through any weak moments (suggested menus and some useful recipes are given below).

4 Tell sisters, brothers and other relatives (especially grand-parents) and also friends who are likely to bring the child presents of sweets. Suggest alternatives (health-food sweets or fruit) or keep a supply to substitute for gifts which have to be taken from the child. Also, when the child starts school leave a supply with the teacher for use as prizes as alternatives to sweets if required.

5 When the child is invited to a party, give her a plate with her own special cakes, sandwiches, crisps, sweets and drink, and explain the situation to the hostess.

6 Ask your local shop to stock foods you need: soya milk, Granose margarine, sheep's cheese – and keep up the pressure!

7 Ask your butcher to mince lamb for you if your child is allergic to beef. Buy game when in season.

8 Cook a few portions for the child and freeze them.

9 When possible, have all the family eat the same food, for example casserole, rissoles, sausages.

10 Don't be afraid to experiment: for instance, substitute soya milk and baking powder for milk and egg. Make 'custard' with soya milk, cornflour and carob powder.

Suggested menus and foodstuffs

Drinks

Use soya milk instead of milk, as a drink and on breakfast cereals. Other drinks which are suitable include soya and banana milk shake, apple juice and 7-up.

Breakfast cereal

Rice has a very low allergic response, and reputable brands of rice crispies do not contain artificial additives.

Bread

This should be either homemade or one that agrees with the child, but if the child is allergic to cow's milk use soya milk for baking.

Butter

If the child is allergic to milk, use milk-free margarine. Granose margarine is a vegetable spread. Kosher margarine is available under different brand names, Tomor being the recommended one.

Jam

Use homemade jams, honey, and pear and apple spreads which contain no added sugar or other additives. Barley malt is also a tasty spread. If the child has a reaction to orange skins, don't use marmalade.

Soup

Practically all packet or tinned soups contain monosodium glutamate, colouring and other additives.

A quick soup can be made from Vecon and tinned tomatoes: liquidize the tomatoes and juice, add a heaped teaspoonful of Vecon and half a pint of water, a pinch of salt and a quarter-teaspoonful of sugar; then bring to the boil and simmer for two minutes. Onion soup is another quick soup.

Vecon is a vegetable concentrate with no additives. Check the ingredients to ensure that it contains none to which your child is allergic.

Meat dishes

Minced lamb can be used to make lamburgers. If the flavour is too bland, add to the meat half a teaspoonful of Vecon dissolved in a quarter-teacup of water. A dash of soy sauce (check the ingredients) also adds a good flavour.

The flavour of vegetable burgers can also be enhanced with the above, and with some olive oil. Vegetable burgers are a product which smell like sausage but contain natural colouring (beetroot) and spices.

Spaghetti bolognese can also be made with minced lamb, served with grated goat's or sheep's cheese. Sheep's cheese can be bought as a feta-type cheese (Greek or French), hard *queso de Manchego* (Spanish) or blue Roquefort (French). Make sure these cheeses are made from 100 per cent sheep's milk. The feta type can be frozen, and it seems to grate better after freezing.

Venison is another useful meat. Deer are susceptible to bovine diseases such as brucellosis and tuberculosis, so make sure you buy your meat from a reputable supplier. The flavour may be too strong for some young children, but it can be disguised in stews, curries and casseroles.

If the child is allergic to chicken, turkey can be substituted. Turkey portions are now available, and these can be fried, roasted or stuffed. Turkey products of all kinds are widely available, and these can also be used in a chicken casserole recipe, or marinaded and served as kebabs:

Turkey kebabs marinade

   1 tablesp. olive oil
   1 tablesp. lemon juice
   1 teasp. cumin
   1–2 cloves garlic
   Turkey leg/breast pieces

The turkey pieces can be fried and then put on kebab sticks with whatever vegetable(s) the child is permitted. Red and yellow peppers make a very good colour display.

Pheasant can be bought in the game season and frozen. These contain no antibiotics as they are free range (even if reared for game). The meat may taste a little dry, so it is best roasted wrapped in tinfoil.

Pheasant with cabbage

Brown a pheasant in about three to four tablespoonfuls of olive oil, then lower the heat and cover the pot, leaving the meat to cook for about twenty minutes. Slice a head of cabbage thinly and blanch for ten minutes. Drain the cabbage and add it to the pheasant. Add seasoning and continue cooking for a further ten minutes. Pour in a cupful (approximately 8 fl. oz.) of plant milk (cream) and simmer for a further five minutes.

Rabbit is another chicken substitute. This can be very tasty in a casserole. Although it contains lots of small bones, which can be a problem where children are concerned, if they are given the right pieces the children will enjoy it.

Rabbit casserole

1 rabbit	*marinade*
2 tablesp. olive oil	1 glass of white wine or Vecon stock
2 cloves garlic	1 small glass of wine vinegar/juice of
3 carrots, sliced	1 lemon
	2 sprigs of thyme
	2 teasp. oregano
	1 bay leaf

Joint the rabbit, cover it with the marinade and leave it for several hours or overnight. Remove the pieces of rabbit, dry them and then brown them in the olive oil. Lower the heat and add the marinade, adding more stock or wine if necessary to cover. Add the chopped garlic and carrots. Simmer for one hour.

Desserts, puddings and party fare

Chocolate pudding. Make up cornflour as instructed on the packet, but using soya milk. Add carob to make a chocolate-flavoured pudding. The cornflour can also be cooked with vanilla to make a white custard.

Jelly. Agar-agar can be used to make jelly, using Ribena (or beetroot juice) as a colouring. Sliced banana or chopped apple can be set into the jelly.

Cream. Planmil, which is a concentrated soya milk, can be used as a substitute for pouring cream. Malsum is a kosher cream substitute, made from palm oil, which can be whipped. It can be sweetened with honey, maple syrup or homemade jam.

Creamed coconut can also be useful here. This is a solid which can be reconstituted with water. It can then be whipped as desired.

Yogurt. Soya yogurt may be made using a yogurt dried enzyme (available in health food shops). Follow the instructions on the packet. It doesn't always work well with soya milk.

Ice cream and lollies. A delicious ice-cream substitute can be made by freezing 'cream' with added raspberry which colours the ice cream pink. 'Cream' can be either Malsum, which includes palm olive oil, and can be whipped (available from kosher shops) or Planmil, which is concentrated soya milk, and is used for pouring. Ice-cream wafers contain E102, so a substitute, such as brandy snaps, may be used instead.

Ice pops and lollies can be made using special containers and freezing diluted Ribena (Baby Ribena contains no additive or colouring), apple juice, orange juice, etc.

Apple crumble

  2 cooking apples
  1 tablesp. brown sugar
  1 teasp. allspice
  1 teasp. cinnamon
  4 oz wholemeal flour
  2 oz white flour
  3 oz brown sugar
  3 oz Granose margarine/white Flora

Peel and slice the apples, put them in an ovenproof dish. Sprinkle on the tablespoonful of sugar and the allspice. In a separate bowl, rub in the flour and margarine, mix in the sugar and cinnamon and spread over the apples. Bake at 350°F for three-quarters of an hour.

When it comes to cakes, check the recipe, substituting soya milk and baking powder for milk and egg where possible (but don't try to make eggless sponges or meringues!). Pastry can be made this way, and Granose margarine can also be used as a substitute. (Viennese pastries are made using an eggless recipe.) You can use the pastry to make either apple or jam tarts or mince pies.

A mincemeat substitute can be made using the following ingredients:

¼ pt water
1 large cooking apple, peeled and finely chopped
4 oz sultanas
¾ teasp. mixed spice
1 teasp. lemon juice
2 tablesp. barley malt

Stew the apple in the water for about five minutes. Add the other ingredients and cook for a further five minutes. Allow to cool before filling the pastry.

Peanut butter biscuits

2 oz peanut butter
3 oz margarine
4 oz brown sugar
5 oz white flour
soya milk

Cream the margarine and sugar together, mix in the peanut butter and then add the flour. If the mixture is too dry (this will depend on the type of peanut butter used), add some soya milk. Roll the mixture out until it is about half an inch thick, cut out into biscuit shapes and then cook for approximately fifteen minutes at 350°F. Allow to cool on the baking tray for a few minutes before turning out onto a wire rack.

Festive occasions

Be sure to have a special treat for the allergic child at festive times: for instance, at Christmas an eggless fruit cake can be made, then iced and decorated. Ordinary icing can be used, and it may be coloured pink with a little beetroot juice (water in which beetroot has been boiled).

Eggless cake

> 12 oz plain flour
> 6 oz margarine
> 6 oz brown sugar
> 1 heaped teasp. bread soda
> 2–3 tablesp. soya milk
> ½ pt cold apple purée
> 4 oz chopped dates
> 4 oz chopped nuts
> 8 oz raisins

Rub together flour and then margarine, add the other dry ingredients. Next add the apple purée and finally the milk. Put the mixture in a greased and lined two-pound-loaf tin. Cook at 350°F for one and a half hours.

Easter eggs. These can be a problem. After many experiments, I have devised an egg which is neither too sweet nor allergic. Using empty grapefruit skins as moulds, cover Rice Crispies with a toffee mixture. When these have hardened, remove mould and pour melted carob drops over the mixture to form a chocolate egg. The shape can be improved by the use of proper moulds.

To make toffee

> 8 oz sugar
> 4 oz golden syrup
> ¼ pint of water

Heat all ingredients in a pot. Allow sugar to dissolve. Boil until little of the mixture when dropped in a bowl of cold water forms a hard ball.

Party treats. Carob Rice Crispie buns may be made by melting carob buttons as one melts chocolate. If carob buttons are not available, melt hard margarine and mix in carob which has been blended with a little water.

Also popcorn can be made at home, using popping corn available from health food shops.

To make popcorn

　4 tablesp. popcorn
　2 tablesp. oil

Put in a pot with lid. Swirl to distribute ingredients evenly. Cover the pot. Heat over medium flame. When first kernel pops remove from flame for one minute. Return to heat. Shake pot until all kernels have popped.

Appendix 8

Useful Names and Addresses

United Kingdom

Hyperactive Children's Support Group
59 Meadowside
Angmering
Sussex
BN16 4BW

Midlands Asthma and Allergy Research Association (MAARA)
12 Vernon Street
Derby
DE1 1FT

The National Society for Research into Allergy
PO Box 45
Hinckley
Leicester
LE10 1JY

Milk Allergy Self-Help Group (MASH)
Mrs A. Camock
4 Queen Anne's Grove
Bush Hill Park
Enfield
Middlesex
EN1 2JP
Tel.: 01 360 2348

National Eczema Society
Tavistock House North
Tavistock Square
London WC1H 9SR
Tel.: 01 388 4097

The Asthma Research Council
12 Pembridge Square
London W2

The Chest, Heart and Stroke Association
Tavistock House North
Tavistock Square
London WC1

The Chest, Heart and Stroke Association
28 Bedford Street
Belfast

United States

Asthma and Allergy Foundation of America
801 Second Avenue
New York NY 10017

National Foundation for Asthma
PO Box 50304
Tucson AZ 85703

Canada

Allergy Information Association
Room 7
25 Poynter Drive
Weston
Ontario

Asthma Information
c/o The Toronto Lung Association
Tel.: (416) 226 1454

Asthma Society
Tel.: (416) 481 9627

Australia

Asthma Association Citizens' Advice Bureau (ACT)
Tel.: Canberra 81 01 85

Asthma Foundation of Queensland
PO Box 122
East Brisbane
Queensland 4169

Asthma Foundation of Southern Australia
13 Hindley Street
Adelaide
Southern Australia 5000

Asthma Foundation of Tasmania
PO Box 18
Hobart
Tasmania 7001

Asthma Foundation of Victoria
2 Highfield Grove
Kew
Victoria 3101

Asthma Welfare Society
249–251 Pitt Street
Sydney
NSW 2000

New Zealand

New Zealand Asthma Society
PO Box 40333
Upper Hutt
Wellington

Republic of Ireland

Eczema Society of Ireland
c/o Mary Inglis
Kilfenora
Gordon Avenue
Foxrock
Dublin 18

Hyperactive Children's Support Group of Ireland
Sarah Nichols
4 Elton Park
Sandycove
Co. Dublin

Irish Allergy Treatment and Research Association (IATRA)
PO Box 1067
Churchtown
Dublin 14

Irish Asthma Society
24 Anglesea Street
Dublin 2
Tel: (01) 716551

Index